METAMORPHOSIS

SURVIVING BRAIN INJURY

To Larry,

Best wishes,

To Sarah.

Introduction

No one wakes up and says, *"By the time the sun sets tonight, I will be critically injured in an accident and left with a debilitating brain injury."*

But that is exactly what happened to me.

November 11, 2010 was perhaps the most defining day of my existence as it was on that fated day that I suffered a life-changing brain injury.

The decision to write this book has been months in the making. By offering what amounts to an insider's view into the world of MTBI (Mild Traumatic Brain Injury) my hope is to help cast a spotlight on what has been called by many *America's Silent Epidemic.*

The CDC estimates that over 1.7 million Americans will suffer a brain injury this year, yet there is a distinct void in real-life information about what life is like living with a brain injury. Practical medical information abounds but real-life insight is almost non-existent.

If you are a health care provider, perhaps this glimpse behind the curtain will offer you new insight as you care for your patients. If you are the family member of someone who has suffered a brain injury, perhaps you will be better able to understand the new and sometimes baffling challenges your loved one faces. Most importantly, if you are someone who has suffered a brain injury and this book has found its way into your hands, know that you are not alone. Please know that there is life after brain injury - a different life, but a life very much worthwhile.

I invite you to join me as I share my journey toward a new wellness. Take my hand, and let's walk for a while. I have quite a tale to tell.

Chapter 1
The Day The Earth Stood Still

"I am fading away. Slowly but surely. Like the sailor who watches the home shore gradually disappear, I watch my past recede. My old life still burns within me, but more and more of it is reduced to the ashes of memory."

~ Jean-Dominique Bauby, *The Diving Bell and the Butterfly*

November 11, 2010 was a day like most others. Little did I realize that by the time the day wound to a close, I would be rushed by ambulance to the nearest trauma center with injuries that would impact me for the rest of my life. There was no sense of impending doom, no feeling of dread, nothing to foretell what the day would bring.

I was more on top of my game than I had ever been. Weeks earlier, I celebrated my one year wedding anniversary to my best friend. My writing career was progressing with recent national publications of my work; my business was strong; my family was healthy and life was good.

Living the dream, I was at one of those places in my life that I have now come to cherish. You know the place... nothing significant is happening and you bask in the ebb and flow of a stunningly normal life.

By day's end however, I would be forever changed. My very soul would be autographed by the grit and asphalt of Main Street. There is nothing pretty about a cycling accident with severe and life-changing injuries. My blood, the very source of life coursing through my veins, was destined to stain Main Street in an odd parody of modern art.

Many people with a traumatic brain injury have little or no recall of the event that changed their life. I, on the other hand, recall the Impact with stunning clarity.

The lasting effects of my head injury on my memory have been among the most challenging, but I'll get into that in much more detail later... if I remember.

The beginning of this chapter of my life predates my brain injury by many years. It's a bit odd to think that my brain injury actually has its roots in diabetes. Never have I read about diabetes being a cause of brain injury. In fact, you might just be privy to what amounts to a medical miracle, but I'll let you decide.

Also worth noting is my propensity to be a bit A.D.D. A month or so after Impact, my speech therapist said something that caught my ear: she shared that those with A.D.D. who have had brain injuries very often jump into the realm of what she called "Super A.D.D."

Suffice to say she was correct.

Both in my writing as well as conversationally, I jump around more than I ever have. Luckily, most all of the time I am able to get the proverbial train back on the tracks and move forward.

The roots of this tale can be traced back to 2007 when I was diagnosed with Type 2 Diabetes. Weighing in at 260 pounds and more comfortable with a Twinkie and a Coke than just about anything else, a trip to my primary care physician confirmed that I was a full blown diabetic; my blood sugar was off the charts, my vision was failing, and I had a veritable wellspring of other symptoms.

"David, take a good look at your feet", my doctor said. "Either use them or lose them." Knowing that

[8]

amputation from untreated diabetes is not uncommon and having an affinity to remain two-footed, I did something not many do. Pretty simple concept: I actually listened to my doctor.

Through the first half of 2007, I got healthy - very healthy. I am a chronic overcomer. Little can or has kept me down for long. Some call it resiliency. I call it stubbornness.

Six months later found my weight down close to 80 pounds. I was in the best shape of my life and very much on top of my game. Cycling thirty miles or so daily gave me back my life. I was always fond of cycling as a child. My diabetes gave me back the gift of loving the ride simply for the sake of the ride. With the wind in my face and the winding road in front of me, cycling remains my undying passion to this day. My story of victory over Diabetes was published nationally and I became a bit of a local poster child for wellness.

I was in better shape at 49 than I was at 29. You could bounce a coin off my calf. Over 40,000 miles of cycling in the short span of a few years does tend to tighten you up a bit.

And life changed abruptly in two ticks of a clock.

The driver who hit me was only 16. I met him and his mom a couple of weeks after the accident, but that is a tale for later. It was quite a meeting. This same young man makes what amounts to a cameo appearance toward the end of this tale, our lives yet again coming together at unexpected and unasked for times.

Local police estimated he was cruising along at between 30-40 MPH when he broadsided me. He never hit the brakes. My accident was of the double-dipping variety. When I was hit from the right, my helmeted head went through his windshield. As the laws of physics are not to be broken, the momentum of his car catapulted me 50' down Main Street where my head impacted the pavement on the left side.

Brains are like Jell-O Gelatin in a Tupperware container. When my head went through his windshield, my brain impacted the inside of my skull in a millisecond, only to bounce back to the other side of my skull. That same dance was repeated when I hit the street giving me the benefit of four internal brain impacts.

Permanent damage to my frontal lobes was diagnosed at a much later date. In fact, a well-intentioned doctor called me "permanently disabled." You'll meet him a bit later.

The impact was so violent that my helmet literally sheared hair off my head. My helmet suddenly became the catcher's mitt for two odd and unexpected items: newly shorn hair and broken glass. In fact, my wife Sarah spent several days following my accident pulling small shards of glass from my head.

There is nothing even remotely attractive about this type of accident.

Two ticks of a clock.

Tick...

Happily cycling on a near picture-perfect November day...

Tick...

Outstretched on Main Street... Broken bones, broken bike, shattered helmet and unable to move. I awaited certain death. Oddly, I was at peace, content with my life. My children would be in good hands. Those close to me knew they were loved. My last words to my wife were "I love you." If it was going to be my time to explore the Next Realm, so be it. Mind you, I was not happy about this possibility but I did have a stunning level of acceptance.

In what amounts to be unbelievable in light of my injuries, 48 hours after my accident, while the events were still fresh, I wrote about my accident. As I was casted from a broken elbow, I painfully and methodically penned my experience, one slow keystroke at a time, using a single finger. Driven by some power within me, some need to chronicle from the start, a journey I didn't even know I was about to embark upon, I did what I've done for years. I put my thoughts on paper.

Chapter 2

Impact + 48 Hours

How long it took me to pen a blog a mere 48 hours after my accident, one painful letter at a time, I cannot tell you. I've read and reread my first attempt to put some order to all that happened, to try to understand. I smile to this day at my innocence, not knowing at that time that more of my injuries were beyond what any doctor could see and were beyond what anyone ever really expected.

Well over a year after my accident, a well respected neuropsychologist added a completely unexpected twist to my recollection of the accident. These days, not much surprises me. His twist did not merely surprise me - it shocked me, as it will you - but the details of this stunning revelation will come later.

I am a writer. In what amounts to an odd twist of fate, while so much has been stripped from me by my accident, my ability to pull together the words to offer in vivid detail the events of my life remains untainted. In fact, the loss of my "emotional filter" since my head injury has given me a voice that was previously buried.

There is very little that I won't chronicle in exquisite detail. The very fact that my voice not only remains, but has clarity heretofore unknown offers me more motivation to share. While so many have lost their ability to communicate from their own brain injuries, my words live on.

Actual blog excerpt from two days after my accident...

"It was inevitable. Sarah & I joked half-heartedly about it for years. On Thursday November 11, 2010 it finally happened. At 3:45 PM my life course was abruptly changed. It was at that moment in time that the car struck me while cycling.

I was broadsided.

T-boned. Blasted into an unexpected and unasked for flight.

Police estimate the driver was doing close to 40 mph when he struck me.

I write, in part, to cleanse my soul. To sort through. To no longer swim beneath. To understand. To try to make sense.

I went through his windshield.

For the first time in my life, I am experiencing true flashbacks. It's like someone splices a scene from Thursday into The Moment, then, as quickly as it plays, someone hits the stop button.

3:45 PM... My favorite band blasting in my MP3 player, my mind trying to find a way to work next Wednesdays show in New York into our busy life. Twenty-two miles under my belt. Sun on my face, smile in my heart. A true state of bliss.

3:47 PM...IMPACT. In a millisecond, everything changed. I was airborne. The most surrealistic experience of my life. The best way to describe it: time "stretched." Though physics would only allow me a few seconds of Superman Flight, my mind's eye made it feel like a full 20 count. There was an odd peace in my spirit as I soared. Flying through the air, maybe living, maybe dying. I watched the road below, and marveled at the composite material. The glitter of mica and the way it sparkled made me think of Disney. I could not believe how long my flight lasted.

And I thought, "it's really gonna suck when I hit the ground."

Fate was kind and stole the memory of impact from me. Closer to the truth- I was knocked senseless.

Flashbulb/strobe light memories came next.

"Call 9-1-1. Call 9-1-1," screamed someone.

"Don't move."

I opened my eyes. Flat on my back, I was incapable of moving.

More screaming.

"Has anyone called 9-1-1?"

I watched bystanders weep. I will be forever haunted by the woman standing by my feet, hand over mouth, tears streaming down her face.

"Always think we get more time..." A line from one of my favorite songs by Third Eye Blind echoed in my head.

As I lay there on the street, I wondered if this was the part of the movie where I would fade to gray and be gone from this life forever. The final act of my life. No encore, no hidden track. Just a fade to gray lying on Main Street. I felt the tears slide down my face and thought of Sarah.

"Call my wife. 205-xxxx. Call my wife. 205-xxxx. Call my wife. 205-xxxx."

I must have said this twenty or more times. Jim, an unknown passerby did just that.

The wail of an ambulance. Rescue vehicles. Lying on Main Street, maybe living, maybe dying.

Strapped to a body board by paramedics. I see nothing but the ceiling of the ambulance. IV's... One, then two needles. My veins accepting their destiny.

"What's your name?" "What day of the week is it?" "What city are you in?" I knew the drill. Making sure somebody was home. Just because my lights were on did not mean I was present.

Listening to the scissors as they cut my cycling clothes off, assessing my beaten and broken body.

Not wanting to be outdone by the ambulance siren, I wailed too.

"We can give you something strong for pain. Something very strong..."

Wanting my wits about me, I declined heavy painkillers.

I was alive.

I bit my lip and settled into a bit of relief brought on by intravenous Advil.

The EMT's called ahead to the Trauma Unit and briefed them.

Finally heeding my constant calls to call Sarah, one the medics in the ambulance called her cell phone. And she followed the ambulance to the ER, her soul mate strapped to a body board in the ambulance in front of her.

Funny thing about being immobilized... you can only stare straight up. As they wheeled me into the trauma center, Sarah's face came into view.

Her eyes swollen. A forced smile on her lips.

"I love you bunny" she said, then, in a heartbeat, she was gone.

I mumbled... "and behold, the face of an angel looked down upon him..." Somewhere, someone laughed.

Trauma Unit talk...

"We need to do a CAT scan... he may have brain bleeding..." I let them know we have two cats and neither would be fond of scanning. Hushed laughing as they jumped into high gear.

You will be spared more of the medical jargon. The final tally: broken arm, mangled wrist, mangled ankle, torn leg muscles, soft tissue damage all over, grapefruit sized bruises and aches I never knew possible.

But I am alive. I can walk, though haltingly.

Already I have changed. I have learned a lot about myself. Strength resided within me that I never knew.

I've been in high emotion since Thursday. Bouts of tears. They say it's normal after trauma.

Still alive.

I've read and reread that blog post perhaps a dozen times since Impact. To this day, it leaves me in tears. As I still cycle thirty miles most every day, several times a week I pass the exact spot where I was hit. There is no apprehension as I approach the intersection that changed my life. There is no low-level panic; no angst or anguish to define the moment. Rather, there is a profound sadness. As I bike up Granite Ave, my thoughts are almost always the same.

"It was on this very section of road that I lived the last few moments of my normal life."

Living with a brain injury is perhaps the toughest road I have walked down, and I've walked more than a few turbulent paths.

The first indication that something was not right happened in the Trauma center as the Deliverers of Miracles worked on my broken body. The nearest well-equipped trauma center was across the state line and what a bustle of activity it was: Doctors, and more doctors; Technicians, and more technicians; a veritable herd of nurses; all working furiously. By this time, I knew I was able to wiggle my toes, bend my legs slightly and feel boatloads of pain. A wave of relief passed through me as I knew my spine was not severed.

Still braced and immobilized, most of what I experienced I saw through my peripheral vision, with an occasional human passing within my limited field of view. I will refrain from any profanity, so I won't have the opportunity to say that I was "scared shitless."

(But I would say that if I could.)

My recall of my first awareness of possible brain damage came with unexpected clarity. Sarah's beloved face in my limited view, she held my hand and we spoke in soft whispers.

And then I was gone.

I could see Sarah above me, her lips moving. But no sound passed from her lips to my ears. Her eyes a mask of worry as she tried to call me back to the present. I lay there; eyes wide open, feeling as if I was being yanked backwards away from reality, like looking down a long hallway. It was a true out of body experience.

And then I was back.

Panic struck as she told the attending trauma doctor of my unexpected hiatus. I was back home in my body by this time, so it was passed off as just part of the traumatic experience of the day and nothing more. It was never recognized as a precursor of the next chapter of my life.

As my condition was not yet known, nor was it known if I would even survive my injuries, a police officer from my town was dispatched to the hospital to take a statement. Standing somewhere in the trauma center, he watched this chaotic scene unfold. As I was still on a back board and unable to see anything other than the overhead lighting, I didn't even know he was there.

With the prior approval of the doctors, he appeared in my limited field of vision to ask me a few questions about the accident. His presence there added yet another layer of surrealism to the events of the day as it was clear that he was there to follow through with the investigation in case my fate was to die.

Hours later, braced and wrapped, I did the unthinkable. As there was concern about brain bleeding, I was told I needed to stay overnight. Not even a smile was offered when I told the attending trauma team that hospitals were for the sick and the infirmed. I was neither and I was going home, against medical advice.

I had enough. Beam me back home, Scottie. Kirk out.

On a side note, having a brain injury can be a lonely business. On one hand, I want to talk about my experience. It is the biggest life-changing event of my life - a veritable game-changer. On the other hand, when you mention a brain injury in most social circles, you are not well received. It is as quick a conversation stopper as talking about say, venereal disease. Everyone knows it exists, but no one wants to talk about it.

Brain injury affects over 1.7 million Americans every year. Called America's silent epidemic and, like most survivors, I choose more often than not to suffer in silence. Silence can help keep already tenuous relationships from completely disintegrating.

Though unknown to me at the time, my new life as a brain injury survivor was about to start. November 12, 2010 was the day the new me was born.

Looking back on life just after my accident, I realize I have scattered memories of the first few months. There were a few milestone events that came to pass that I remember with clarity, but most of those early weeks are lost. With the benefit of hindsight, I now realize that this is perhaps one of my greatest blessings. I have one sliver of a memory from Thanksgiving Day 2010 and virtually no recall of the first Christmas after I was hit.

Looking back on pictures that were taken during the 2010 holidays, I can be seen smiling, looking a bit beat up, still casted and braced, but very much alive. Such is the nature of my new life. By all outward appearances, I have recovered. The breaks and bruises have been corrected by time, but it's the unseen injury that has become the biggest challenge of my life. In fact, it is safe to say that my accident has become singularly the most life changing event of my life.

I look back on those holiday photos and wonder where I was. In body, I was part of the ebb and flow of life, talking to Sarah, working on the business of healing, wrapping my mind around my physical injuries and how to get well as fast as possible. The holiday photos prove I was there! But any and all recall of having the pictures taken, of what we did on Thanksgiving, of who I saw on Christmas, has all been erased from my memory.

Brain injuries are not immediately recognizable. It was not until early 2011 that the full extent of my brain injury would become evident. Thinking that much of what I was experiencing in the weeks after my accident was the result of the trauma to my body, I discounted some of the early warning signs.

Having checked myself out of the hospital the night of my accident, I was handed the phone number of a local orthopedic office to attend to my breaks as well as the phone number for a neurologist to assess any potential brain damage.

The orthopedic experience the next day was quite typical: all black and white. Read the x-ray, pinpoint the breaks, cast me up and send me on my way - all quite clinical and predictable.

As my orthopedic visit was under 24 hours after my accident, my fingers had just begun their own transformation process. They were slowly mutating from fingers to small sausages as my damaged arm and hand continued to swell.

Long before my accident, I learned one of life's most important lessons: "Wear the world like a loose garment." As a very predictable rule, material items don't have a lot of hold over me. Cars come and go. I've been privileged to own a couple of homes in my life. Not concurrently, mind you. It is a very safe bet to assume that I won't be driving my current vehicle in twenty years and, I probably won't be in the same home, or wearing the same clothes.

Material things come and go. There is an immense spiritual freedom in understanding this simple concept.

But there is one material item that I fully expect to have with me until the day I die: My wedding ring. I fully expect to have possession of this until I draw my last breath.

The orthopedic doctor took one look at my hand and said quite simply that my wedding ring needed to come off immediately. In typical David form, I balked at his request. Smiling and delivering his next message with purely clinical candor, he replied, "If your wedding ring stays on and your hand continues to swell, you may lose your finger."

Not wanting to emulate Frodo Baggins and walk through the rest of my life explaining away a lost finger, we tried to heed his call. Handing us a small vial of some type of lubricant, he was quite clear that he'd be back in a few minutes and expected the wedding ring to be removed.

"If you can't get the ring off, I'll have to cut it off."

Sarah and I sat there in stunned silence.

Just fifteen months prior to my accident, Sarah and I were married at a seaside wedding ceremony on the coast of New Hampshire. On a sunny August day that would have made any tourism department absolutely green with envy, we exchanged our marriage vows outside under a warm summer sun.

The backdrop to our ceremony was the Atlantic Ocean. Sailboats with full white sails passed behind us under a cloudless blue sky. Both of us barefoot, toes deep in green grass, we were surrounded by people who loved us and who shared in our joy. I had Sarah's wedding ring custom made to forever nestle into an antique engagement ring she still wears. My wedding ring was made to match her unique set.

There was no way it was going to become yet another victim of that fated day, so we went to work. My hand literally bathed in lubricant, we worked and worked at getting it off my swollen finger. One millimeter at a time, it made its way off my hand. The pain was close to unbearable but, the prospect of forever losing the most sacred possession I own carried even more pain.

Though never spoken aloud, I would have traded a finger to have my wedding ring left intact. Happily, I left that day with both.

You could almost hear the walls of the exam room exhale as the ring left my finger. For the next month, Sarah wore two wedding rings. The ring that I placed on her finger in the presence of friends and family, and my own ring, for safe keeping until I was fit enough to wear it again. A month or so after the accident, it made its way back onto my hand. My accident has robbed me of the memory of its return, but I wear it to this day.

And, so ended the orthopedic visit. I hobbled out of the office, a cast on one arm, a boot on my foot, my wedding ring on Sarah's finger, and words from the doctor letting me know my expected recovery time. Right on cue, I was walking again on two feet in about a month and in pain for six months from my broken elbow. Truth be told, when the doctor said it would take half a year for my elbow to heal, it didn't bother me a bit. I prefer the land of the concrete, the finite, the predicable, to the realm of the unknown in a heartbeat. If he told me it would be a year even that would have been tolerable. At least it set my expectations.

Funny thing: At the six month anniversary of my accident, my elbow did indeed stop hurting.

From the orthopedic office, I was off to see the neurologist. I was immediately impressed by the concern and apparent proficiency of the young neurologist. At least ten years my junior, his approach spoke of kindness, compassion and concern.

He assessed my records, reviewed my CAT scan from the day prior and conducted what is called a MoCA test. The Montreal Cognitive Assessment, or MoCA test, is a brief test administered to see if there are any cognitive problems. I passed the test with flying colors a mere 24 hours after my accident. Letting me know I had successfully dodged a bullet, he patted me on the shoulder as my wife and I left his office letting me know how lucky I was. He extended an invitation to call him if there was ever an issue, and wished us both well.

Little did I realize that a few short weeks later, I would be in his office, terrified and confused.

Chapter 3

Many Meetings

Through the pain and fog of the weeks following my accident, there were events that came to pass that are virtually impossible to forget. For many years, I held the steadfast belief that nothing happens by chance. No matter how painful, all happens for the greater good. As Sarah still reminds me constantly, "the curse will become the blessing."

The young man who drove his car into me did so at a fortunate location. I was struck down a mere two blocks from our town's main fire station. A week after impact, it was time to pay a visit to that local fire station.

Still looking like I had recently been run down by a car, sporting a foot brace, arm in a sling and presenting a look that spoke of shell-shocked, Sarah and I took the trek to the Main Street Fire House. A bit of an aside here: I bake. I love to bake. On Wednesday nights I meet up with some friends at a local college and come bearing brownies every week. My Wednesday night friends gobble up close to 300 pounds of my brownies a year.

Walking through the front door of the fire station, I came bearing brownies. Well, technically, Sarah was carrying them, but I was still able to whip out a one-handed batch of brownies in advance of our trip.

Why go to the fire station so soon after the accident? It's pretty simple. A number of our local firefighters, rescue workers, paramedics and more were all part of the team that got me off Main Street USA and on my way to the trauma center. How could I not take some time to thank them personally for their service to our community and look them each in the eye and offer a sincere and heartfelt thank you?

Our local fire station has a small entry room with glass windows that divide the dispatch area from a small reception area. Behind the glass, a staffer asked how he could help us.

"I'm the guy that was scraped up off Main Street last week, and I want to say thanks to the guys who helped me," I blurted out. Still unaware of my brain injury as my body was working through the healing process, already my disinhibitionism was beginning to show through.

We were buzzed though to the back room of the station, where a kitchen area borders a dining table. Akin to being backstage at a concert, I expect this was not an area frequented by civilians. The Captain on Duty entered the room. We chit-chatted lightly as the room filled with our local firefighters. One by one, they filed in. Looking around, there were close to a dozen young men who come to work every day, ready to risk their lives in service to our community.

"Can I ask which of you was there the day I was hurt?"

First one hand went up. Then another followed. Then another. And another. All told, ten or more of the firefighters and paramedics in that room were on the accident scene that fated day. The Captain shared that because the accident was so close to the station, pretty much the entire staff came over to assist, with many walking the two short blocks to the accident scene. It was an emotionally charged and powerful moment.

And it drove me to tears.

I made it a point to look each one of the young men in the eye, and offer a heartfelt thank you. Sarah, ever-present by my side, offered her thanks as well. This was not the last time I was to see this group of life savers.

Though one of the largest communities in New Hampshire, our town still maintains a small-town feel in many respects. Neighbors wave to neighbors. Local business owners know and remember their regular customers, and politicians still shake hands in our annual Christmas Parade.

Still blissfully unaware of the extent of my brain injury, three short weeks after my accident, our annual Christmas Parade proceeded down Main Street. Still braced, bruised and casted and, trying to recover from my physical injuries I decided to attend the 2010 parade. Sarah by my side, my mom and dad there for the occasion, we staked out our territory in front of our local library to partake of the afternoon's festivities.

Truth be told, parade watching remains one of my favorite activities. From the street vendors wheeling carts of overpriced toys to the ever-present balloon merchants, there is high energy and much happiness and ever-present anticipation in the air.

Our town has a very predictable parade format. Every year, the parade is led by a phalanx of firefighters and rescue personnel. Carrying up the rear of the parade is Santa, usually perched high atop a fire department ladder truck. Between this parade Alpha and Omega, marching bands, dancing schools, and homemade elementary school floats are the standard fare for the day.

In the years immediately following 9/11, even when parade participants were still out of sight, you knew of the impending approach of fire and rescue personnel by the applause in advance of their arrival. 9/11 had brought together so many of us in a spirit of patriotism and, first responders were the face of real American heroes.

In a show of deep respect for their service, parade watchers would get up from their chairs and applaud loudly as these brave men and women passed by. Sadly, this tradition faded out a few short years after 9/11, though I still make it a point to stand and applaud loudly as they pass. I expect I always will. As

I have had the chance to see these workers of miracles in action, my respect for their selfless service has deepened over time.

Unable to stand for long periods of time after my accident, I sat roadside in quiet anticipation of the day's events. What was supposed to be a joyous day was about to become one of the most emotionally charged memories of life after my accident, though I knew it not at the time.

The firefighters and rescue personnel leading the parade numbered twenty to thirty that year. I stood in a show of well-deserved respect as the firefighters passed. While marching, they wear much of their protective gear. Several carried fire axes. As they are marching directly behind the American flag that leads the entire processional, it is a visually stunning image.

As they passed my wife and me standing in roadside homage to their dedication and service, it happened. I saw one of the firefighters point to me, say something to his marching companion, and offer a broad smile and wave of recognition. As others within their ranks looked over to see who was attracting their attention, more and more arms arose all waving at me.

And they smiled.

I knew from my recent trip to the firehouse that not every story has a happy ending. Such is the nature of life. Car accidents, domestic violence, house fires, all of these can and occasionally do end in the loss of life. Yet there I stood, roadside and alive, a living testament to the actions of these selfless souls.

By the time they had passed me, close to half of them were smiling and waving. Tears welled up in my eyes. How do you really thank someone who places their life on the line to help others? The parade kept marching, as all parades must do, and they passed me in what was most likely under a minute. Yet, that minute has created a memory I will cherish for a lifetime.

I fell into the chair behind me, awash with emotion. My wife and mother were both there in an instant asking if I was okay. As emotionally charged as that chance meeting with my rescuers was, it was followed up by an introduction I would never have expected.

Life is truly stranger than fiction.

Sometimes I feel like a soul from another time. These days, everything seems so rushed. Everyone seems so intent on rushing from one unimportant task to another. Ruefully, I admit I can get caught up in this as well, though my pace is noticeably slower since my accident.

I had a call to make. During the early weeks after the accident, I was filled with a deep appreciation for all who help save my life, who interceded either directly or indirectly. I carry that appreciation with me to this day.

From the paramedics on scene to the Trauma Center doctors, I was told repeatedly that my helmet saved my life. This is one of the common sense truths that deeply affect me.

Helmets do indeed save the lives of cyclists every year. I am living proof.

Giro, the manufacturer of the helmet that saved my life, was on my short list of folks to contact. Like most of the larger corporate entities, they have a telephone call center to handle inbound calls to their corporate office. While their typical customer service representative probably runs the gambit from general inquires to product specific questions, the call that I placed one morning a few weeks after my accident was far from a typical call I suspect. In fact, I can most assuredly say this.

The intent of my call was simply to request the corporate address to send a thank you letter. Truth be told, I do not recall the name of the young woman who took my call that fated day.

"I need to make sure a thank you letter that I will be sending ends up where it's supposed to," I let the unsuspecting recipient of my call know.

Eager to help, she asked about the nature of my letter.

"You see, a Giro cycling helmet saved my life a couple weeks ago. From initial engineering to production and ultimately to distribution, a helmet that bore the Giro brand prevented my certain death."

There was a long pause as she pondered what to say next. I ended the brief moment of silence by telling her my story, most likely in a bit more detail than necessary.

By the time I wound down, I was again in tears, happy to be alive to tell my tale. She was crying too as she shared that mine was the first "thank you for saving my life" call she was part of.

Though I suspect Giro helmets have saved countless lives, and no doubt others have called, it was a first for her and for me.

Like my trip to the Main Street Fire Station, it would be unforgivable for me not to express a heartfelt thank you. These days, when I ride, I still wear a Giro helmet. Yes, there is a fierce sense of brand loyalty. More importantly, I can attest from real-world experience that they have a good product. Is this an unsolicited endorsement? You bet it is.

My early meetings with so many were about to come to a close. I was soon to meet the young man who was behind the wheel of the car that hit me.

Still trying piece together exactly what happened when I was hit, and unclear how I could possibly have been broadsided by a car on Main Street, I had a couple of conversations with the officer conducting the investigation.

While the investigating police officer concluded that the accident was a true "no fault" accident, the insurance company representing the young man who was at the wheel conducted their own investigation. The final result of the investigation by the insurance company allocated 51% of blame of the accident to me, 49% to their policy holder.

As I was, in their opinion, the majority shareholder in the events of that day, they used it as their basis to deny any claims related to the accident. Bodily injury, hospital bills, and follow up care were all to be my responsibility. Here in my home state of New Hampshire, unlike many other states, a 51% at-fault judgment allows the insurance company to simply walk away as their policy holder holds the minority share of the blame.

When I asked a representative from the insurance company if they used an independent investigator, I was told quite directly that it was someone on their payroll. I was cordially wished the best of luck and the conversation was abruptly terminated by the insurance company representative.

The purpose of this book is to illuminate the path that many brain injury victims walk. Having been told that I was on my own still brings forth anger. I have never been one out looking for an "easy pay check." It's against everything I believe in.

In conversations with a couple of local attorneys, the accident falls into what is called a "right of way" violation. Very challenging to prove in court, I was told by members of the legal community to concentrate more on getting well. There are many injustices to the brain injured, but living as a victim bars the path to real recovery. I aggressively move around most anything that stands between me and wellness.

The investigating officer let me know that my bike, heretofore impounded, could be picked up at our local police station. Still unable to drive, Sarah drove me over to pick up what was left of my bike. The investigating officer, only a few years older than one of my own sons, let me know that the family of the young man who hit me had been desperately trying to reach out to me.

This young man, not knowing what shape I was in, was completely devastated by the accident. Privacy laws prevented our local PD from releasing any information about my condition to his family. The officer politely asked if he could provide the drivers family with my phone number.

As a father of four sons, the "dad" in me kicked into high gear and I let him know that releasing my number would be fine. At the time, I expected nothing more than a possible conversation, and nothing more.

We came home from the police station that day to our phone ringing off the hook. It was the mother of the young man who hit me. We spoke for ten to fifteen minutes on the phone. Her son, rendered almost non-functional since the accident, was alternating between bouts of uncontrollable crying and what looked like depression. His family was on the cusp of getting him outside help.

And she asked if we could meet him.

Not thinking before I spoke, I asked her to put him on the line. It was purely an act of impulse and one that I do not regret to this day.

Here was another human being who was suffering. I held, at least in part, the key to emotional freedom for him. Being a dad with sons, my mind kept wondering what I would have said had this been one of my own sons.

I let him know that I was alive. That I would recover. And that they are called "accidents" for a reason. Trying to inject a bit of humor into the conversation, I said to him, "You are a lucky kid. Odds are that you will only hit one cyclist in your entire lifetime. Two important points to consider: At least you got it over with early in your driving career and, better still, you had the wherewithal to hit a nice guy."

He laughed and asked if we could meet.

His mom came back on the phone, and we decided to meet a few days later at a bit of a neutral spot: the parking lot of our local high school.

My mindset before meeting the young man who forever changed my life was not one of nervousness. It's important again to reiterate that at the time of our meeting, I was blissfully unaware of my brain injury. Battered and beaten, bruised and sore, I was still most likely in shock as my body was just beginning the long, slow crawl toward what would become my new normal.

As I was still held hostage by an arm in a sling and a booted left foot, Sarah drove to the local High School for our meeting. Of all the high emotion events that followed my accident, meeting the driver of the car that struck me was, by far, the most emotionally charged.

We pulled into the high school parking lot. It was a quiet, albeit short ride from our house to the school. To this day, Sarah carries a lot of anger toward him. I've never made her wrong for this, as we all have our paths to walk. We move forward through life not at a pace defined by others, rather, we come to grips with events that come to pass in our own time. I have no right to make my schedule hers. We all find our own truths.

We got out of our cars at close to the same time. It was still a struggle for me to move at that time, but I was out and on my feet... um... on my foot, in no time.

We stood there, face-to-face, eye-to-eye for a few seconds in a bit of stunned silence. He was a young man tormented for weeks about the fate of someone he had yet to meet. There I stood, high emotion right under the surface, looking at the one whose actions caused so much pain, so much strife, so much anguish.

And the clock ticked for a few more seconds as we sized each other up.

What I recall most clearly is the sense of innocence he projected. No arrogant demeanor, no punk attitude. In front of me stood a young man who was clearly hurting, who had experienced sleepless nights and tormented days, not knowing whether I was capable of walking, of talking, of carrying on even the most basic of life's functions.

His red-rimmed eyes stared up at me, almost hauntingly. I did and said what any dad would do.

"Come here and let me give you a hug."

In hindsight, it was the most apropos thing I could have said. I offered a heartfelt, though one-armed hug, and the conversation opened up. As noted already, being a dad of four sons offered me what amounted to the best "on the job training" I could ever have hoped for. I was presented with what amounts to a very unique and God-given opportunity. I looked him in the eye and let him know that in no uncertain terms, everything was going to be fine.

Time is a funny thing. With the passage of time, new perspectives are gained, new insights emerge. I have often thought what I might have said to this young man had I known the extent of my brain injury at the time we met. How would I have reacted had I known that the very course of the rest of my life was changed the day of my accident? That I was to have struggles unimagined.

Truth be told, had I knowledge of what was going to come to pass my actions that day would not have changed. Somebody much wiser than me once said that resentments are like wanting someone else to die, but you take the poison. To this day, I wish nothing but happiness and peace to him.

Life happens. Accidents happen. And life invariably does go on.

We stayed in the parking lot for close to half an hour. Sarah and I, the young man and his mom, talking

[47]

under a waning winter sun. His mom asked if it was OK to stay in touch. They even made our Christmas card list that year. Though 2011 would bring unforeseen and difficult challenges, I was grateful simply to be alive. Not every cyclist lives after meeting metal at close to 40 MPH.

Sarah and I got into the car to head home. The young man came bearing chocolates, flowers and other sundry treats that helped soften my heart. Those who know me know that I have a vicious love of all things sweet. Though my life is much different today, chocolate still resides quite high on my list of all-time favorites.

The short ride home was a bit on the quiet side. Sarah was lost in her thoughts while I was grateful to be part of helping this young man let go of something that he might have carried for a lifetime. I don't think about him often anymore. Our paths converged the day of the accident and diverged the day after our meeting. He makes a cameo appearance toward the end of this tale, but you'll read about that later.

My hope is that he doesn't think about me often as well, as odd as that sounds. He is a young man with a full life ahead of him; a life brimming with promise, opportunity and unfulfilled dreams. As time passes, my normal life seems like a distant dream. To spend too much time looking backwards is to slow my progress moving forward.

But so much of life is two steps forward and three steps backwards.

Unknown to me at the time was that I was about to take a few steps backwards - very, very big steps.

Chapter 4

Welcome to the Discovery Channel

Over time, it became apparent that this was a tale that needed to be told. As noted, millions and millions of Americans live with the silent stigma of head injuries. Add to this all of the lives touched by those directly afflicted and it's safe to say the number of people impacted by traumatic head injuries can be conservatively measured in the tens of millions.

My original intent was to simply offer a chronology of events, offering insight as to the journey I continue to walk. I will be taking an occasional breather, however, along the way, to interject a bit of how my life is today. To offer insight as to what life is like living with a brain injury.

I have also made the very difficult decision to hold back nothing. I do this in an effort to fully reveal the ongoing struggles of living with a traumatic brain injury. Some close to me may be saddened or even shocked by my revelations, but there is no need to be. I am alive.

In the grander scheme of life, my fate could have been dramatically different. I could have died that day. Life bound to a wheelchair could have been my destiny. Yes, though harsh to some, the hand of fate spared me a potentially heavier blow.

I have come to realize that since my brain injury, life is increasingly fascinating. In fact, life since my accident has been the most fascinating of my entire existence. Fascinating in what I fondly call a *Discovery Channel* kind of way. By this I mean that it would be an amazing 60 minute TV special to watch. But to live it, to experience it all first-hand - this is something I would not wish upon anyone.

Just recently, for example: I went partially blind for a while. Yet another layer of amazement sets in as I am able to simply state this as if talking about going out for a coffee. Just before bed one night, I lost the vision in my right eye. Now you see me, now you don't. Trying to work through my newfound blindness, I settled down and tried to read from my Kindle.

Little did I realize at the time that in addition to my newfound blindness, a case of extreme light sensitivity struck at the same time. When I powered on my Kindle, it was akin to a 50,000 watt spotlight shining directly into my brain. That was about all it took for me to call it quits for that night.

The very next night, I lost half my vision in the same eye at bedtime. From the horizon line down was simply gone. I dared not try to turn on my Kindle based on my experience of the night prior, I simply went to bed.

In a day and age where access to more information than exists in all the world's libraries is virtually at your fingertips, I tread very carefully. In researching my back-to-back temporary blindness episodes, Google revealed that vision problems, up to a couple of years after a brain injury, are not uncommon.

Once I read that nugget of information, my research ceased immediately.

Yes, I could have conducted exhaustive research, looked at all the possibilities of my blindness, weighed the pros and cons of each scenario, but I chose not to. What would I have accomplished? Having a brain injury is hard enough by itself. I steadfastly avoid the deliberate manufacture of outcomes that may never be part of my own reality.

At roughly the same time my world, albeit temporarily, became dark, I wrapped up my last session of neuropsychology testing. In its simplest terms, this testing is designed to evaluate specifically what areas of my brain are damaged as well as to offer an assessment of what types of functioning, cognitive and otherwise, are negatively impacted by my accident. Upon completion of my testing, it was time for The Great Reveal; the meeting with the doctor, Sarah, and me, to go over the final results from my neuropsychology testing.

My neuropsychologist shared that I had tested in the bottom 5% of folks for complex problem solving abilities. He also noted that my testing showed me to be in the lower 20% based on verbal memory. Simply put, I am capable of wonderful, engaging, thought-provoking and highly animated conversations - conversations that I will all but forget within a few minutes. I'll get into more detail about The Great Reveal a bit later.

We can add one more event to the trifecta of the last couple weeks. In addition to my blindness and completely disheartening comments by the neuropsychologist, I was also diagnosed with Post Traumatic Stress Disorder. My PTSD symptoms are pretty much textbook perfect. Larger crowds now cause extreme angst and anxiety, where in my past life I loved being completely immersed in humanity. Sudden and unexpected noises startle me at a level never before experienced. The sound of a siren wail from a fire truck or ambulance more often than not brings me to tears.

And there are the nightmares; Vivid, terrifying and unending. To give you a real feel for what my life can be like after dark, I have included, as a bit of an afterword, a couple of short stories about the nature of my nightmares.

Life After Dark, presented at the end of this book, will offer you a bit of chilling insight as to the inner workings of a damaged brain.

Between my lack of any real meaningful sleep, living with a mind that tormented me after dark, and all the other challenges that presented in the weeks prior to my neuropsychology testing, I found myself in an emotional and life-threatening tailspin.

Strike that.

I found myself in full-blown crisis mode.

Several months after my accident, when the nightmares became unbearable, and medications prescribed did nothing to abate my night terrors, I sought out the help of a holistic care provider. I found myself sitting in her office, eyes red-rimmed from tears and lack of sleep, letting her know that I had reached the jumping off point. My life had gotten to the point of no longer being even bearable.

Afraid that I could not go on much longer in the state I was in, and too afraid to die, my back was against a wall. I was going to be dead within a week, or as a better scenario, perhaps incarcerated where I would not be allowed the benefit of my belt or shoe laces. For the first time in my life, I thought about having myself institutionally committed before self-harm became part of my fate.

Such was the point of complete and unadulterated despair I found myself in a full 14 months after my accident. Sitting on the couch at my therapists' office, unable to hold back the tears, I put all my fears out on the table. Akin to sitting in emotional nakedness, I had no option but to be 100% candid. By being open about my problems, I can be more receptive to solutions. When suicide starts to look like a real solution to life's problems, then all perspective is indeed lost. Hope is gone. Darkness surrounds and the light of all reason is snuffed out.

And I thought of Sarah.

My mind, no longer my friend, whispered to me. And I almost believed the lies. It told me that if I were to remain alive, I would torment her with twenty or more years of worry. Yet if I died, within a couple of years, she would come to grips with her loss and move on to a happy life.

My mind told me that my own children no longer needed me. As adults, or close to adults, I was an unnecessary part of their lives. And I fantasized about how I would die and the words I would have for God when I finally had the chance to see Him face-to-face.

If this isn't crisis, I don't know what is.

Sitting in my therapists' office in historic Exeter, New Hampshire, my soul was bared like no other time in my life. Raw with fear and emotion, I shook as I shared with her my state.

A woman 15+ years my senior with a small frame and a big heart, she listened to me. I cannot stress the importance of having someone impartial to talk to. Sarah is my wife, but she is not my counselor. Without the ability to openly share my fears, in a judgment-free zone, you would not be reading these words as I would be yet another statistic; yet another one of many who succumbed to the long-term challenges of living with a brain injury. My accident would have killed me. Not at the point of impact. No, my death, a direct result of my accident would have occurred more than a year after impact.

As I wound down, she got up, crossed the room, and clasped both my hands in hers.

"David, you need to make a pact with me. If you ever reach the point where suicide looks like a viable option, you need to call me first."

She stared me straight in the eyes and would not let go. The clock on the wall ticked off a few seconds, then a few more. The silence became a palpable being in the office.

And I agreed.

And my fate was sealed. No harm by my own hand.

She also dropped a bomb.

"If I have that type of concern for you, you KNOW what I have to do."

We talked for the next ten or fifteen minutes about action items I needed to take to help improve my sleep, to get over this most recent hurdle. I left her office feeling 50 pounds lighter emotionally. Better still, hope was rekindled as I had a new plan that just might lessen (or even eliminate) the ceaseless nightmares.

Again, to frame all of this in a bit of proper context, these events came to pass at over a year since my accident. At fourteen months I was in worse shape than I was at six months after my accident. Such is the nature of life with a brain injury. It's wild and untamed, waiting to ambush you at the next turn, so ever-present vigilance becomes a way of life.

Chapter 5

An Unexpected Diagnosis

Many years ago I heard a short, witty saying that I carry within me to this day...

"If you want to make God laugh, make plans."

In the first month or two after my accident, I made plenty of plans. Enough, I suspect to have God belly-laughing. My plans were quite simple, actually. I planned to get well. And I planned to move on in my life, chalking up the experience of that fated day as a day to remember. I was not naive. Rather, for the first month or so after my injury, as my body healed, I lived in the land of blissful ignorance.

Truth be told, I wish at times that I was there still, living in the land of Bliss. To this day my PTSD nightmares still bring me back to that child-like state at bedtime where the dark scares me. Where the fear of what might be coming soon terrorizes me; where the end of the day brings no solace.

On the surface, Thanksgiving and Christmas 2010 passed uneventfully. Turkeys were cooked. Gifts were bought and wrapped. Our tree was trimmed and holiday celebrations and customs continued.

But I have almost no recall at all of these events. For many years, I have had a passion for photography. Though my brain injury has robbed me of so much, my passion for photography remained unchanged. I have a veritable wellspring of photos from both Thanksgiving and Christmas that immediately followed my accident.

Photos of the holidays, I have. Memories of those days, however, I have not.

Pictures abound of me smiling, holding Sarah's hand, smiling in our kitchen, and pictures of family. There is enough visual proof to sway the most skeptical of juries. Yet if you asked me to share any details of those first holidays, you will be met with a blank stare.

I will continually revisit the fact that life with a brain injury is surrealistic. Up is down, left is right and, at times nothing makes any semblance of sense. This is especially hard for someone like me who likes order and routine. Major memory challenges continue to this day.

As I attempt to piece together those early months, I will do so taking good faith guesses at the timing of some of the more noteworthy events that came to pass.

It was early January 2011 that it became apparent that not all was well. I was still living with an undiagnosed brain injury. Life was about to get very strange very fast. I was enjoying the last remnants of living in the bliss of ignorance. I was about to have the rug pulled out from my reality, but knew it not.

And it all started with a batch of brownies.

A creature of habit, I have been baking brownies most every Wednesday for close to a decade. As noted earlier, meeting some of my close friends on Wednesday nights at a local college had become a bit of a custom. My weekly trips to the college found me with fresh baked brownies to bring to the gang.

I know the recipe by heart. With hundreds of pounds of brownies leaving my kitchen every year, it's hard not to. Four eggs, one cup of oil, half a cup of water are just part of the familiar list. I can recite it in my sleep.

Yet one fated Wednesday in January found me in my kitchen, staring at the bottle of oil, with no idea what to do. I know it now as a cognitive challenge. At the time, however, I was left totally confused. I stood in my kitchen with a box of brownie mix in one hand and scratched my head with the other. I read and reread the directions over and over again and had no idea what to do; no idea where to start.

And I was afraid.

Let's face it; reading directions from a brownie box is not really rocket science. Prep work that normally took 5 minutes required close to half an hour of emotionally and mentally exhausting effort.

For the first time since my accident I was scared. Actually, scared is an understatement. I was completely terrified. For weeks after my accident, I think that I knew, at some primal level, that something was not right. My broken body went from screaming in daily pain to dull aches. The sun rose and the sun set and weeks passed.

Repeatedly I said to Sarah the same words, "I do not want to be *that guy*."

Early on, she gently asked, "What guy is that?"

And I let her know that in no uncertain terms did I want to be, "the guy folks would say was never the same after the accident." My soul probably knew before my conscious mind that all was not well, that there were more to my injuries than just my breaks and bruises.

It was time to call back the neurologist - the very same one who congratulated me for dodging a bullet with brain damage. My inability to recall how to do a very familiar task like baking, coupled with close to two months of incessant tinnitus, robbing me of any real peace, was enough of a requisite to get me back to the doctor's office.

A few days later found me sitting in the same chair in the same office that I occupied the day after my accident. In a hauntingly familiar repetition of the day after my accident, my neurologist again conducted the same MoCA test. For my second consecutive time, I passed with flying colors.

A bit of a side-note is order as well. I have learned from personal experience that brain injuries can be elusive to diagnose. Both MoCA tests came back within the realm of what is deemed normal. My CAT scan and EEG both came back normal. On paper, I was a healthy 49 year old man. But we all know there is so much more to life and a meaningful, accurate diagnosis than what shows up on paper.

I sat there, Sarah at my side, and shared my newfound challenges with the doctor. Unlike my shell-shocked condition the day after Impact, I had a wealth of information to present to him. From my cognitive challenges and vivid nightmares to the incessant ear ringing, from my memory lapses to my newfound friend, constant vertigo, I did my best to describe my symptoms accurately, without any real fanfare.

In typical doctor fashion, he took notes. How long we were there, I can't tell you. As I wound down, he looked at us both and presented his diagnosis.

Calling it one of the most clearly defined cases of post-concussive syndrome he had ever seen, he went on to admit that, yes, I did indeed have a concussion at the time of my accident.

And that I did indeed suffer a brain injury.

You might wonder how I reacted to his new and changed diagnosis. Again, mindful that this was the same doctor who had proclaimed my luck in completely avoiding a brain injury just a couple of months earlier, that day he sat bearing news of an entirely different nature. The pendulum now swung in an entirely different direction.

My response to the new diagnosis consisted of a couple of simple questions.

"When will I get over this?"

"How long will it be until I feel normal again?"

Staring at me long and hard, and with firm conviction in his voice, he let me know that within a year, I'd be back on top of my game, back in the Big Chair, ready to rock n' roll as if nothing had ever happened.

Truth be told, that didn't bother me a bit. Even had he said two years, I would still have walked out of his office a happy camper.

I beat things. Always have, always will.

If the well-versed, highly educated doctor said I was going to be normal within a year, then it would be so.

As I was two months post-impact, I was left with only a small ten month window.

There was an air of excitement as Sarah and I walked out of his office for the second time. Sure, I had a new diagnosis. But I also had a timeline, the firm assurance that I would get better and my current suite of challenges would, in the not too distant future, be behind me.

There was also a prescription for Meclizine in my pocket. You know that feeling you get when you are leaning a bit too far back in a chair and you find yourself ready to fall backwards, but at the last moment, you catch yourself? Your heart races as you know you almost took a header, but were spared the humiliation of a fall. Well, I lived with that same feeling, almost incessantly, for weeks after my accident. Vertigo, loss of balance and dizziness are common among brain injury survivors.

I was also prescribed Amitriptyline for the chronic and debilitating headaches I was experiencing.

Prescribed for headaches, one of the side effects of Amitriptyline is suicidal thoughts. Though buried deep in the prescription documentation, I was never told to be mindful of this.

I left the doctor's office with hope in my heart and a prescription for disaster in my pocket. A prescription that almost turned me into a statistic a few short months later.

Leaving the neurologist's office the day after impact, I never thought I would be back. Leaving the same office a couple months later, I had that same feeling: I was going to be moving forward toward reclaiming my life.

But Fate had other plans for me: Plans much darker than anything I could conceive of.

That light at the end of the tunnel was really a train.

Chapter 6

Friends Fatale'

The Internet is a funny place. We live in a day and age where we have instant access to more information than exists in every library in the world, right at our fingertips. Many years ago my stepson was diagnosed with cancer. Only thirteen at the time of his diagnosis, Sarah and I learned firsthand that life is often hard and unfair. His lead oncologist at the time cautioned Sarah and I about reading too much online about the type of cancer he had.

As only the voice of experience can do, she let us know that we could spend a lot of time reading about challenges we would never face and battles we would never be part of. We wisely heeded this advice. My stepson beat cancer and we were spared months, perhaps even years of mental anguish.

This experience came reeling back to me full-circle with my newfound diagnosis. Early on, I made the conscious decision to look for information only on a "need to know" basis. Sometimes however, living on a "need to know" basis revealed information I wish I never knew, but was oddly grateful that I had stumbled across.

Having a relatively healthy social life before impact, I had many well-wishers ask me how my recovery was progressing. In the first few months following my accident, I did indeed look like I was run over by a car. My injuries were quite blatant and apparent to anyone who saw me.

Though now living with a new diagnosis, I was still blissfully unaware of the social stigma attached to brain injuries. More interesting still was the fact that I really did not understand what disinhibitionism was all about. Disinhibitionism is the removal of the social and mental filter that prevents you from really speaking your mind at inappropriate times. Disinhibitionism affects many with an acquired brain injury.

When well-intentioned friends would ask how I was progressing in my recovery, I thought nothing of answering honestly.

"Thanks for asking, <insert former friends name here>. My breaks and bruises are healing nicely. But man, oh, man, a brain injury is such an interesting experience."

Somewhere early on I read that a person with a brain injury loses on average, over 90% of their close friends within a year of the injury. Though shocked by that number, it was NOT going to happen to me. I had supported many friends throughout the years and they would support me. That was, or so I thought, the way life is supposed to work.

At the one year anniversary of my accident, over 90% of my closest friends were gone.

With time comes a bit of wisdom: Wisdom born of real-world experience. Mention brain injury in casual conversation and you immediately make most people quite uncomfortable. No one likes to look at their own mortality. Brain injuries do just that. They are an "in your face" reminder of how fragile life really is. And it makes people feel uncomfortable.

And human nature is what it is.

They avoid the source of discomfort.

They avoid me.

Always one to make lemons from lemonade, it really is time to interject a bit of humor. You see, you can parlay this knowledge to your advantage in ways totally unexpected.

Have you ever been at your local market, perhaps a corner store, and run into someone you'd rather not see? Perhaps the nosey neighbor; maybe a friend you had a falling out with. You know the scenario. With a brain injury, those uncomfortable chance meetings just got a lot shorter.

"Hi David. Nice to see you. How are things?"

Letting a slow smile spread across my face, these days I have been known to answer, "other than a recent traumatic brain injury, life is pretty good."

You know that old saying about yelling FIRE in a crowded theater? Well, a well-delivered candid reply like that has virtually the same effect. It can stop a conversation and clear a room in a ten-count. In fact, it can be predictably funny.

Over time, many people, some I've known for years, simply drifted away. I understand why. And oddly, it doesn't bother me as much as you'd think. I would prefer not to be a source of discomfort. If it means that I have to become invisible to some, so be it. That is one I'll take for the team. And I'll gladly spare someone an awkward moment.

But there are a lot of people I miss.

The price of admission into the Land of the Brain Damaged is steep. There is a lot of carnage along the way and the body count is high.

The road can get very lonely.

Very lonely.

Chapter 7

Together We Can

It was a short four months after my accident when I got a call that was to be one of the first turning points in my journey. For the first few weeks after my accident, before my "official" brain injury diagnosis, I met with a speech therapist at a local rehab hospital. Ironically, my speech challenges had yet to manifest, so by mutual agreement, our visits ceased.

Several months later, as the breadth and depth of my injury began to manifest, I called the therapist and asked for the "self-pay" rate. (I've got quite a tale to tell about insurance companies a bit later.) As it was still very early in 2011 and my sky-high insurance deductible had not yet been met, any hope of ongoing speech therapy was going to come if I could afford it on a cash basis.

As the local rehab had a record of my insurance coverage and policy information, they quoted me a rate close to $200 an hour. In what amounts to a bit of an irony, if I was uninsured, the rate would have been $85 an hour. In a conversation with one of the admissions staffers to see if opting to receive care on a self-pay basis was feasible, I was told that if the insurance company found out that I was paying only $85 an hour, they would adjust their payments to the hospital to reflect the lower rate.

I became a revenue-loss risk to them. Such is the power of the larger insurance carriers over institutions that are tasked with offering care. At $200 an hour, my choice was to pay my mortgage or to go to therapy. My house is still deeded in my name, so you already know the choice I made.

In the course of one of my conversations with a staff member at the rehab hospital, I was told about a newly forming support group for "high functioning" brain injury survivors. The first meeting was to be held in April of 2011 and I was a perfect candidate for the group.

In over the half-century that my life has spanned thus far, I've seen amazing wonders. I've seen all four of my own sons take their first breath. Nothing can hold a candle to watching lava flow down Kilauea at night and roll into the sea in billows of steam. From sunsets over the desert to simply watching Sarah as she sleeps, I have experienced joys unimagined.

But like any other human being since the dawn of time, hardship has reared its head repeatedly. From the unexpected loss of family members to a bankrupt business, some heavy blows have fallen. This does not make me unique. It simply makes me human. I carry no hard feelings or resentment about any of my challenges or difficult experiences. In fact, at a deeper level, I can appreciate them as they strengthen me. As steel is tempered and made stronger by fire, so have the fires of my own life, including my brain injury, made me stronger.

Long ago I learned an important life lesson: Problems carried alone are problems doubled while problems shared are problems cut in half. Looking back over the most difficult challenges in my life, those times that I was part of a peer group of others with similar experiences were dramatically easier than those times I tried to go it alone.

Such was my life experience and mindset when I learned of the new MTBI Support Group.

I am blessed in that the rehab hospital is only a short ride from our home. In fact, the ride over is under five minutes. Arriving for the first meeting ten minutes early, I found an easy parking space, grabbed my notebook and started a new part of my journey I am walking to this day.

A bit of a perspective check is in order. Until that first meeting, I have never knowingly met someone with a brain injury. My understanding of my injury was just beginning and my awareness of my newfound limitations was growing. Virtually all of my knowledge up to this point in time was presented to me by well-intentioned doctors, by books I had read, and by information I had found online.

I can recall that first meeting like it was yesterday. Walking into the conference room, I was both anxious and excited. Having no idea what to expect, I was a proverbial blank slate when I arrived. And life was about to again change.

A couple of folks sat at a conference table. After poking my face through the door and seeing what appeared to be just a couple of staffers engaged in conversation, I mumbled something about having the wrong room. As I started to exist stage left, one of the attendees called to me.

"If you are looking for the brain injury group, you've found it."

Truthfully, I'm not sure what I was expecting. Wheelchairs? People with visible challenges? I was completely both out of, and in my element at the same time. I can look back on it now and smile as I "look" normal - just as my newfound friends did.

Over the next few minutes, the room slowly filled with people. People who looked just like you and just like me. It's not called America's Silent Epidemic without just cause. By the time the meeting started, there were a dozen of us there, brought together by a shared tragedy, and now bound together by an unasked-for life experience.

The facilitator took a couple of minutes to explain a bit about the group, talked about the direction the group may go in, and started the dialogue by asking each of us to share what happened to bring us there. The stories that unfolded that night were breathtaking.

Stunning events had come to pass for everyone there that night.

One by one, we shared what happened.

From the young college student who had hit a tree while skiing to tale after tale of auto accidents, I sat there spellbound. There was even a cyclist like me who was injured by an errant driver. So much for being unique!

Yes, the causes of the injuries were as different as wildflowers in a meadow. But what shocked me were the tales of life after tragedy. Here were a group of people who shared challenges I had never before heard articulated by another soul. From speech problems to memories that no longer functioned, from incessant tinnitus to chronic exhaustion, I was among those who knew of these things not from reading about them in books, but from actually living life with a brain injury.

Initially scheduled for an hour, our first meeting went over by about ten minutes. Simply put, no one wanted to leave. There was an immediate sense of comfort, a palpable sense of peace that came from simply being in the presence of souls with similar fates.

Though I only had a five minute ride home after the meeting, I made the decision to take a long-cut and not head straight home. My head was spinning. I was no longer alone in my challenges. That night I met people who have long since become my friends.

And I cried.

The water works started before my key even found my car ignition. I cried like I had never cried before. The pent up fear, frustrations, anxiety, apartness and more all came out. Red rimmed eyes met Sarah at the door that night. She looked at me, said not a word, and embraced me.

We still meet once a month at the hospital. There have even been get togethers at some of the homes of the regular members. And I've never missed a meeting.

I cannot overstate how critical, how cathartic and how vital to my own recovery these meetings have been. And they've grown. We have newer members who drive (or are driven) from 20 - 30 miles away to be part of this cherished group. Though I have quite intentionally tried to forego giving any direct advice, I am going to deviate a bit here. If you are a brain injury survivor, please find a group. You'll thank me for it.

Over the last year, we've had guest speakers, hours and hours of face-to-face sharing and, a new Facebook Group lets us stay in touch between the monthly meetings.

And yes, there is a perennial box of tissues at our meeting, often making its way up and down the full length of the table at every meeting.

Chapter 8

The Land of the Endless Summer

From suicidal thoughts to lost friends, you've already caught a glimpse of life post-impact. Sometimes life throws a curve ball at you so unexpected, so utterly surreal, that you simply cannot help but to be stunned. Such is life after a brain injury.

Some of my symptoms are quite unexpected, and many of the events that have come to pass since my accident are equally as surrealistic.

Take, for example, my new inability to feel cold. Since Impact, my ability to feel cold has all but disappeared. Never having been overly fond of winters here in New England, at first glance, this may sound like a quite a blessing.

Like many of my long-term symptoms, the awareness that something changed, that something internal shifted, came slowly over time. There was no ah-ha moment, just a gradual realization that something was different; that my new normal had just shifted again.

It was a sunny day in March of 2011. Like I have for many years in March when the weather cooperates, I decided to wash my car in the driveway. A bucket full of suds in front of me and a garden hose by my side, I looked the part of most any weekender partaking in giving my car its ritualistic bath.

Basking with the sun on my face, my body slowly healing from the accident 5 months prior, I noticed longer than normal stares from folks driving by our home. Living on a busy corner, rubberneckers come with this territory. Folks watching what kind of flowers we plant, eyes glancing over as the lawn is being cut, it's all part of life on a corner lot.

But there was something different that day. Very different.

The stares were just a little longer. Cars passing by at a fraction of their normal speed. Like I had done hundreds of times before, I was washing my car in shorts and a t-shirt. No shoes on my feet, my footsteps marked by soap suds in my driveway. This was not, however, a typical car-washing spring kind of day. You see, it was sunny day, but it was not a warm day. The thermometer topped out at only 38 degrees, though I knew it not.

My ability to feel cold had shifted. Sometimes there is no sensation at all when it's cold. Sometimes I feel cold like pain. There is no sensation of any temperature change. Rather, my arms, legs, hands and feet hurt in response to cold.

Odder still, sometimes I feel cold as the color white. This is difficult for me to describe as it defies traditional logic.

I've developed a fascination for TV shows about the brain. Not an obsession, mind you. But if something catches my eye on those rare occasions that I watch TV, and it hits close to home, I watch it.

I recently saw a show about a brain injury survivor. He took a jump into a shallow pool and the resulting impact left him in the same club I'm in. As he slowly recovered, something unexpected happened. Post Impact, he was able to play the piano like a concert pianist. His brain injury catapulted him into the unexpected realm of being a piano virtuoso.

It was fascinating as he went on to describe how he "sees" notes as blocks that flow in front of his field of vision. He simply plays what he sees. He "sees" notes, and I often "feel" white instead of cold. As I watch the purported experts on TV, and continue to work on my own recovery, I am still amazed at how little is understood about the inner workings of the brain.

Losing the ability to feel cold is actually a thrill, but it does require me to take precautions. One of my new adaptive strategies is to dress by the thermometer and forecast, and no longer by what I feel. This is especially true on my 30 mile bike rides as I need to make sure I don't put myself in harm's way by under or over dressing.

Chapter 9

Out of the Frying Pan and Into the Fire

You might think there was an air of sadness or fear immediately after being diagnosed with a brain injury. Nothing could be further from the truth.

Knowledge is power. In early 2011, I had a concrete diagnosis and a timeline to get back to normal. Unlike the quiet drive home from the police station after picking up my bike, the ride home from the neurologist's office on diagnosis day found us both animated and hopeful.

There was no longer any mystery about what was wrong with me. Yes, my symptoms were quite pronounced, but why wouldn't they be? I was, after all, broadsided by several thousand pounds of metal. Though pronounced, the young neurologist still saw no sign of anything to be alarmed about. My symptoms, he assured us, would abate. Life would soon return to normal.

Armed with my newfound diagnosis of Post Concussive Syndrome, I carefully ventured out to the Internet on a fact-finding mission. There is a stunning amount of inaccurate information online. There are pages and pages of conflicting information at every mouse click.

Having a background in technology with information gathering being part of my profession, I discounted much, read even more, and grabbed on to a few nuggets of information that I found to have a feeling of legitimacy.

And I found the Traumatic Brain Injury Survival Guide (www.tbiguide.com) by Clinical Neuropsychologist Dr. Glen Johnson. From WebMD to a wide range of sites offering clinical and personal experience, The TBI Survival Guide quickly became my primary source of meaningful and practical information about my new condition.

Unlike the neurologist who both diagnosed my condition and assured me that in a matter of months, I would be "normal" again, Dr. Johnson shared a fact that helped me beyond measure.

"I've never really met anybody who's claimed to have recovered 100%," he touts in his book. This, after treating many patients over a period of years. It's still surprising how little this bothered me. As I've said before, the truth will set you free.

It is unquestionably better to have a realistic truth than false hopes. Best to have an accurate True North to point my recovery compass at, than to wander through life hoping that somehow, in some way, things would change. Today I do my best to simply accept that "it is what it is" living life with brain injury. I was not going to hop from doctor to doctor, hoping for a magic fix, for the magic mix of medication and therapy that would restore me back to the normalcy I once knew.

This small fact was a game-changer for me.

If I was never going to get back to 100%, then damn it, I was going to get as close to it as I could. Life passes quickly. Too quickly. I made the decision to do everything within my power to get as well as I was capable of. I might not be able to get back to 100%, but I still call the high 90's a passing grade.

My quest toward wellness began.

By this time, I was back on my bike again. In fact, I had been since early January. One of my ongoing challenges - a challenge that still haunts me to this day - is chronic mental exhaustion. In fact, I have not been able to work on a full time basis since my accident. By early to mid-afternoon most every day, my mind simply says, "all done." From that point on, the hope of any further productivity for that day is pretty much gone.

As so much of my new life involves the use of compensatory strategies to make up for what I've lost, I decided to use this deficiency to my best interest. While many brain injury survivors experience both mental as well as physical exhaustion, mine was limited to the emotional weariness only.

While I was unable to put together a couple of back-to-back productive thoughts when emotional exhaustion hit, I was able to hop on my bike and cycle for a couple hours. I am grateful for this as not all who suffer a brain injury fare as well.

Thus a brand new chapter of my post-accident life began to unfold. I started eating healthier and committed to at least 30 miles a day on my bike. Thirty miles, day in, day out.

For a couple of months after Impact, I was overcome by a new and quite delightful challenge: I craved jelly beans. Yes, my sweet tooth had grown by leaps and bounds. It's all too easy to pack a few pounds on the waistline by succumbing to a Jelly Belly addiction. While I'm sure there are 12 Step Groups for Jelly Bean addicts, I made no effort to search one out. I was content with my new obsession. C'mon, it's jelly beans we are talking about here. How bad can they really be?

My neurologist found this newfound passion to be both humorous as well as scientifically grounded in fact. Hypothalamus damage will actually cause sugar cravings. Not only was I now a closet jelly bean fiend, but it was also explainable by medical science.

No sadness here, just bring me another bag of Tropical Punch Jelly Bellies!

Tough decisions had to be made. Cutting back on my Jelly's was a start. Daily cycling was on my short list as well. Realizing that by 2:00 PM, I was all but useless at my desk, but still able to push out the miles made me redefine my days. My new schedule began to take form, to take shape. Work from 7:30AM - 2:00PM, then off for a 30 mile bike ride.

At some point, I would not be surprised to see a scientific study touting the connection between driving highly oxygenated blood through your system for a couple hours a day and faster recovery from an MTBI. A couple hours of cardio every day can't hurt, and may help.

Plus, it filled the 2:00 PM void. I was able to walk away from my desk, essentially brain dead and useless at that time, and still move forward doing something else that would drive me toward wellness.

As the first winter of my recovery was also the winter of record breaking snowfall here in New England, I did the unthinkable. Please don't judge me. Yes, I, who thrived with the wind in my face, resorted to an indoor cycle. From a practical standpoint, cycling on the streets of New Hampshire in the midst of what was turning out to be the winter of the century was not practical, not safe, and certainly not conducive to a happy marriage.

You might be wondering as well what it was like getting back on a bike after my near death experience. We've all heard that you need to get right back on a horse after a fall. But it was more difficult on a bike. I'd like nothing more than to say it was a piece of cake; that I jumped back in the saddle and cycled off into a golden sunset.

My first attempt as a ride was a mere 40 or so days after my accident. My arm was in a short cast and I decided to try some laps on a street adjacent to ours. A small oval loop with little, if any daytime traffic, seemed like a good place to start.

Did I tell you that I have never claimed to be the leader of the pack with common sense?

It was a bad choice to make. Fifteen minutes later, I was home, casted arm throbbing and feeling like it was probably not the best thing to do.

Sarah agreed. Heartily.

These days, my riding is quite different than it was before Impact. Whenever possible, I stay on quieter roads. Roads that pass cow pastures and corn fields are my top choice.

Traffic scares me at some times and terrifies me even more of the time.

Hopeful that the neurologist was right, I innocently and quite naively thought the worst of it was over. I had classified a brain injury in the same category as most any other injury. And why wouldn't I? As this was a new experience for me, I had no prior experience, no internal knowledge base to draw from. I was living in uncharted territory. Like healing from any injury, my recovery would have a beginning, middle and an end.

Today I have come to say what most brain injury professionals say, that my recovery will go on for as long as I have a heartbeat. Very much a marathon and not a sprint.

As you will continue to see, life with a brain injury is unpredictable. While my new life is often three steps forward, two steps backwards, it is also often five steps backward with no forward progress at all.

While my new commitment to getting well, as well as I could, would put me in tip-top shape from the neck down, I was about to find out one of the harsh realities of life with a brain injury. You can have the physiology of an endurance athlete, and still struggle with unforeseen challenges.

From my January 2011 diagnosis until my emergency trip to the neurologist two short months later, I did my best to adapt to my new normal. I've long since learned that the goal is no longer victory over brain injury. Rather, my goal is to coexist with it. It will be with me until the end.

I can fight this fact, or I can choose to live with it.

As brain injury touches every part of my life, from my work professionally, to friendships, to my relationship with my wife Sarah, it is equally important to keep it all in perspective and to not let my life become defined by living life as a brain injury survivor. This is perhaps the most difficult of challenges. It had become the biggest issue in my life, but I could not let it overshadow the fact that I still had a life to live, kids to feed, a mortgage to pay and responsibilities to meet.

Akin to learning to live in new skin, I did my best to bob and weave as my brain injury pummeled me with new and often surprising blows. From the never ending tinnitus to vertigo that still forces me on occasion to grab hold of something stationary lest I fall over, I moved forward, one day at a time, through a life that was unfamiliar at best, uncomfortable most of the time and, more often than not, completely exhausting.

There were some unexpected and exciting consequences as well. And life is truly stranger than fiction. I became a human snow globe.

And what, exactly, does that mean?

Snow globes have long been a holiday favorite of mine. You know what I am talking about: those serene, wintery landscapes captured inside a round glass globe. Simply shake the globe and the snowscape changes with every shake.

The snowflakes never leave the globe. The exact number of flakes never changes, yet the landscape that they produce changes every time the globe is given a shake. So became the landscape of my mind. Every snowflake was a memory. My Impact had the effect of shaking the snow globe of my mind. Memories that should have been on the surface were buried deep. While snowflake memories that were long buried were suddenly, unexpectedly and sometimes delightfully on the surface.

And a strange new occurrence started to happen. I would recall events, sometimes decades earlier in my life, as if they were only days old. I could describe, in exquisite detail, the kitchen of the home I grew up in over 40 years ago.

Faces of friends that I knew in my teens and twenties popped into my mind as if they had never aged. I could tell you about a particular event that happened in 1977 as if it was just last week. Ask me however, about how I had spent the earlier part of that very same day and a blank stare would be my reply. My day-to-day memory fell to pieces. In fact, it is still shattered.

One day, I had a crystal clear memory of one of my best friends from high school. We grew up in the same town, went to the same private high school and held jobs with the same local employer. Yet like so many others, we drifted apart as we got older.

Until my accident.

After that particular snowflake of a memory presented, I did a quick Facebook search and found him. We exchanged a few emails and had lunch the very next week. We still stay in touch and go out for an occasional lunch.

I can say with absolute certainty that this friendship would not have been rekindled, had it not been for the odd quirks of my memory since the accident.

In the first six to nine months following my brain injury diagnosis, I struggled to adapt to living in my new normal. Much of it was uncomfortable. Not mentioned before, I was also living with debilitating headaches as part of my new life as well. You get what you get and play as best you can whatever hand fate deals you. I am fortunate. My headaches were akin to someone driving multiple ice picks into my brain simultaneously. The blessing is that they were short-lived, typically lasting under a couple of minutes.

Call them Houdini headaches if you like, as they disappeared as if by magic.

But nothing would prepare me for what I was about to experience. I was on the cusp of an experience so profoundly frightening, it almost defies description.

February 2011 passed. Winter was behind me and March, with its longer days, was here. For an avid cyclist like me, March and Heaven are synonymous. Not too hot, not too cold, flowers sprouting at every turn, greener lawns and blue skies. March is perhaps my favorite of all months as it signifies the end of winter.

Like I had most every day for weeks before, I hopped on my bike, looked at my watch and planned for a two hour bike ride. Such was my commitment to getting well, five minutes into my ride I stopped to double-check my watch and got the shock of my life.

In my mind's eye, only five minutes had passed. I was only two blocks from my house. Well within where I might be five minutes into my ride.

But my watch said otherwise. Over two hours had passed since I left home. My odometer on my bike had spun up to 30+ miles as well, and I had virtually no recall of the entire ride.

Two hours of time had been permanently erased from my memory. Like a Star Trek Vulcan mind wash, my memory was wiped clean. As I was only minutes from home, I pedaled like the wind. Terrified and confused, I pulled into the driveway. Sarah came out, took one look at me and knew something BIG had happened.

And I was psychotic.

Somewhere between the time I "woke up" and when I arrived home a couple of minutes later, I had become convinced that everything I saw was a dream; that none of it was real. I had the unwavering belief that I was in a coma laying in a hospital bed, my mom by my side, waiting for me to wake up.

As Sarah approached me, I grabbed her hand and held it in mine. I turned it palm up and ran my fingers across it, marveling at the degree of detail my mind was capable of creating as I lay hospitalized and unconscious. The color, the softness of her skin, the stunning reality of my dream.

My eyes and hands wandered for the next couple of minutes. Sarah has said I kept asking if everything was real. Looking at trees in our yard, cars in the driveway, flowers in our yard, I was certain that this was all created by my mind in an effort to keep me going as my time in my imaginary coma passed.

She led me into the house by the hand. I showered, climbed into bed and slept for hours.

And the next day, we were back at the neurologist's office.

It was not supposed to unfold like this. Over time, I was supposed to be getting better. That's how things work. You get hurt, time passes, and you get better and move on. I've been doing that for my entire life. Not so with the human brain.

In the night that passed between my most recent episode and my next-day doctor's appointment, I took a bit of time to jump online. Fear gripped me like fear I've never experienced. I could taste it. Fear caused me to read a little too much, to dig a little too deep. I was concerned that I had some type of seizure while I was riding.

Chapter 9

Unexpected Shopping

Sitting in the same exam room that I was in the day after the accident took on a new element of urgency as I shared with my neurologist the events of the day prior.

He did something so completely unexpected, so completely surreal, that it caught me off guard.

He scratched his head.

By circumstance rather than any virtue, I've developed an understanding of brain injury that only comes with living with it. More of a laypersons viewpoint, I can tell you as much about life with a brain injury as most professionals can, though I can offer what amounts to an insider's point of view. Like a perverse backstage pass to a bit of a human freak show, I can tell you about the challenges I face not because of any literature I've read, nor clinical work I've done.

I live in this reality now. My first life ended on November 11, 2010. It was stripped from me in a violent and unexpected twist of metal and fate. I hold no bitterness, but so much of me died that day. My new life as a brain injury survivor began that day as well.

The Alpha and Omega of my life.

I was ordered to undergo an EEG and MRI as soon as possible, as there was concern of a secondary bleed in my brain. I had unexpectedly jumped back in to discovery mode again. Whoever could have predicted on that fateful day months earlier that I would be forced by circumstance to shop for my own medical care? Our ultra-high deductible health insurance, coupled with the fact that it was still early in the calendar year, forced me by circumstance to become an advocate for my own health care.

We were put in the unexpected position of going shopping. Shopping for what? Why MRI shopping, of course. Suffice to say, MRI shopping was an eye-opening experience. Our insurance company had a list of MRI providers on their website. It fast became a call-list for Sarah as she methodically worked her way through the providers, calling each to inquire about their self-pay rate.

The results were nothing short of astounding. For the exact same MRI test, a high cost of over $4,000.00 was offset by a low of $780.00 - all for virtually the same test on comparable MRI equipment. We had decided early on that a four hour drive for testing was worth saving a couple thousand dollars. We had even given consideration to driving to Canada as we are only four hours from the Canadian border. This, we knew, would have been an overnight trip. But again, if an overnight trip shaved a couple of thousand dollars off the cost, it was a worthwhile investment in time.

Yet again Fate looked kindly upon us. On the lower end of the cost scale was an MRI provider only ten miles from our home.

Over the next few days, I had an MRI, an EEG, and then what would quite surprisingly be our last visit to my neurologist.

It was close to two weeks later that we had a sit-down with my neurologist to go over the test results. Both the MRI and EEG came back clean. It is very common in brain injuries to have damage at the molecular level. In my case, though it was very clear that there were ongoing problems, all clinical testing came back clean. In my new life, I have met many other brain injury survivors whose testing came back just as mine: Normal on paper. Far from normal in real world, practical experience.

The course of my treatment abruptly changed. It was time to bring in the "Big Guns." Yes, my neurologist marched me over to see the head doctor at his practice. I know now that the neurologist I was seeing was a junior practitioner at this office, though I knew it not then. He had very clear concern in his eyes when he said it was time for another set of eyes, a set of more experienced eyes, to look at all that was going on with me.

Sitting in the Top Doc's office down the hall, he took a few minutes to consult with my doctor and read my files. For the next thirty minutes, he questioned me, took copious notes, questioned me some more, took more notes, fired a question or two at Sarah, took even more notes. Then he presented his diagnosis. Quite certain that I had dodged yet another bullet and not had a seizure, he called the two hours of lost time an incident of Global Transient Amnesia.

I love non-technical analogies. It helps to convey concepts in ways understandable.

Imagine having a great digital camera in hand and going out on a picture taking expedition. Things catch your eye and you snap pictures. If it's a nice digital camera, perhaps you even take a couple of videos.

Imagine as well that your batteries are brand new. The view finder works like a charm. Even the flash goes off as it should. All appears to be working perfectly on this imaginary photo shoot.

But what would happen if you had no film in the camera? Or if there was no memory card where there was supposed to be one? On the outside, all would look typical. Snapping away, you would look like most any photographer. But without film, you would have no record of your pictures.

And so it was with my mind that day.

For a couple of hours, I had virtually lost the ability to lay down any new memories. My camera was working just fine, the batteries were fully charged, but someone forgot to put a memory card in my head. I have had numerous similar events, though nothing as long as the two hours that were unexpectedly removed from my life.

It's troubling. It's scary. There is no way to predict it, nor is there any way to avoid it. Stranger still, if circumstance puts you in my path while this is happening, you would never know. My "camera" looks perfect. We could have an engaging conversation. Perhaps we would talk about current events, discuss politics or the like. I could even get into my car and drive away quite safely. Yet I would simply have no recall of the meeting. Yet another of the odd quirks of life with a brain injury.

In addition to the newly diagnosed Transient Global Amnesia, he went on to confirm that I was suffering as well with a very pronounced case of Post Traumatic Stress Disorder. The nightmares were continuing full throttle at that time and we could now add PTSD to my list of new friends.

Keep in mind that all this new information was being presented over three months post Impact.

There has been a push by many professionals to re-categorize brain injury as a chronic condition. It's a safe assumption that insurance companies will fight this to the bitter end. At the time of my accident, I was a classic case of living life as an under-insured person. Our health insurance policy, carried through Sarah's employer, was more of a catastrophic policy as we had to pay thousands of dollars out of pocket for my care.

As this was now March of 2011, our high deductible had reset and we had essentially no coverage until we hit the high deductible.

And we learned.

We learned that you must become an advocate not only for the quality of your care, but that it was critical to master the business side of the process. Medical challenges are the number one cause of bankruptcy in the US today and we were determined not to be part of yet another statistic

The price of a brain injury transcends simply the initial accident. There are ongoing medical bills and care required to this day, as well as loss of wages that will continue through the rest of my life. I entered Into repayment arrangements with many of my early caregivers based on what I could afford to pay. In many cases, these arrangements will continue for years to come.

By early March, it was clear that any return to full-time work was not going to be happening. Thankfully, I had a rainy day fund that I contributed to for years prior to my accident. As I am self-employed, I jokingly called my emergency fund my long term disability fund, never knowing how close to the truth that would be.

The junior neurologist walked us out of the office that day. For the first time since I had been seeing him, he looked uncomfortable.

And he dropped a bomb.

"There is nothing more I can do for you," he shared. He proceeded to pull one of his business cards out of his pocket. "See? Right here on my card, what you have is not within my area of expertise."

Had I not heard him say that and been there, I never would have believed such a thing could happen. He shared that he might have the name of a Boston doctor at one of the larger hospitals who may be able to help me.

The doctor and staffer spent a few minutes looking for the Boston doctor's name. Unable to find it, he let us know that he'd mail us a copy of the complete medical records and the name of the doctor.

One thing I have not lost is the ability to judge sincerity. It was a brush off, plain and simple. Walking back to the car, I said to Sarah that we were just dismissed.

Game over. Move along.

Always one to look at the positive, she assured me that we would get the new doctor's name, my medical records and, we would move on.

Two weeks later, when no records or doctors name arrived, Sarah reluctantly agreed with me. As the doctor was quite clear he could do no more, there really was no need to ever call him back. In one respect, he did us a favor.

Yet it also felt like we were abandoned. Here was a doctor that I liked, that I trusted, that I believed, who dismissed me with the wave of a business card and a curt goodbye.

Sarah summed it up best when the records still had not arrived a month later.

"It looks like we are on our own with this."

Chapter 10

I Lied

It was a simple question. It was an even simpler lie.

"How are you feeling, David?" she asked.

"Feeling just fine, Mom. Thanks for asking."

I am not surprised by how easy the lie fell off my lips. It's become all too common for me to lie when well-intentioned people ask me how my recovery is going. Sometimes people lie to weave a web of deception. I avoid that like the plague. Other times, people lie for protection.

Lies of *deception* are vastly different that lies of *protection*.

Lies of protection are far more common that you might think. Just ask any parent who has uttered the words, "Santa Claus is real." This lie, present in the childhood of so many people, is keenly delivered to help preserve the sanctity of childhood. Childhood passes all too quickly and many caring parents lie to their children to preserve this innocence for as long as practical. Childhood is fleeting. All too soon, the realities of life as an adult come rushing in. Offering this untruth helps contribute to all that is and can be magical about being a child.

While it may not be prudent to tell a sixteen year old that Santa really exists, sharing this same fact with a five year old is not just commonplace, it's expected.

Sometimes we lie to our children to protect them. Sometimes we lie to our parents for the same reason. To offer protection. Protection from worry, protection from harsh truths that may inflict emotional pain. We may lie to our parents because they are loved. In an odd irony, it is that same reason that they used in sharing some untruths to us as children.

Brain injury places a barrier between people. No one really wants to talk about it. No one wants to see their own mortality, their own vulnerability, in the hand that Fate dealt another member of the human family.

As my social circles got a lot smaller after a life-altering event like my brain injury, I find myself becoming more protective of the precious friendships I have been able to retain. And yes, sometimes that means having to say I'm OK, when, in reality, all is not well at the ranch.

It's a tightrope walk at times, deciding in a millisecond how much information to share when someone asks. Even within my closest circle of friends, I can all too often simply utter an insincere, "I am doing better," to avoid bringing brain injury into the conversation.

I've even intentionally steered the conversation away from this topic so slickly that most don't even notice.

Most never notice, except Sarah. She calls me out on it pretty much every time. Her one-liner remains timeless.

"Nice conversation change."

I cherish those who have remained by my side through what has become the toughest chapter in my life, and fully understand why some have stepped back. There is no anger. No resentment and really no unhappiness.

No one really wants to be the source of discomfort. I would much rather bring joy to those close to me than create an environment of ongoing concern.

There really is something cathartic and freeing about writing. My true voice, untainted by what others may think, shines through. I can share my joys, my sorrows, my fears under the illusion that it's just me, my keyboard and my monitor. Though I know otherwise, it's still an immensely personal experience.

And it's time for another confession.

As just about every day winds down and Sarah and I climb into bed for the night, like pushing the snooze button on an alarm clock in the morning, my hand reaches out nightly on autopilot to activate the white noise machine at my bedside. Though there is a wide range of sound choices, options like waterfalls, waves crashing and even real white noise, I prefer the soft sound of summer crickets. Summer has long been my favorite season. As my tinnitus has stripped away my ability to hear heat bugs and in most cases, crickets as well, I have come to love this infusion of sounds that comforted me in my former life.

With the sound cranked up on the white noise machine, though artificial, I can again hear the wondrous sounds of summer crickets. Without this simple device, the freight train of sound that roars endlessly through my head becomes overwhelming and unbearable. Thank God for this small technology-driven miracle.

There are times that Sarah will look over, see me just staring at the ceiling and ask me a simple question. "How are you doing?"

I see the genuine concern in her eyes. I feel the weight of her worry in her voice.

Most of the time, I share openly about where I am. About what may, or may not be troubling me. I love her. She deserves as much honesty as I am capable of.

But on rare occasions, I lie.

As the passage of time is, for the most part, no longer discernable to me anymore, in what seems like a three-count, I hear her breath become deep and I know she's drifted away to sleep. To her own safe place. A place free from worry.

And I stare at the wall. My hands at times gripping the bed sheets as yet another overwhelming wave of vertigo hits me. Bed spins similar to what I experienced in my college days after a night of too much of the college life; with a big difference. These bed spins strike me while I'm stone cold sober.

I lay there and stare wide-eyed wondering if tonight is going to be yet another night with the PTSD nightmares. A night where yet again, I wake up covered in sweat, screaming. Sarah, by my side, gently trying to pull me back to reality. To safety.

In this quiet time, the enormity of it all hits me hard. There are no distractions. Often, the last thing I feel is a tear running down my face as I continue to mourn the loss of my old life.

Chapter 11

Living Like Tom Hanks

In 2000, Tom Hanks was cast as the unlikely sole survivor of a FedEx plane crash. In the scene immediately after the plane crash, Hanks is desperately trying to escape from the sinking fuselage.

The cinematography by director Robert Zemeckis is simply brilliant. As Hanks swims through the sinking plane, you can hear soft ocean-like sounds. Bubbling and gurgling noise as the air escapes the sinking plane abounds. Akin to what you might hear in an aquarium, the audio track is muted at best.

As Hanks has to survive, he breaks free of the plane and swims to the surface.

As he breaks the surface, a scene of utter chaos unfolds with flaming jet fuel and a still spinning turbine of the jet engine visible. It's not the stunning visuals however, that touch my tale. It's the audio chaos.

In two ticks of a clock, the big screen soundtrack goes from relative quiet to ear-popping screaming sounds and screeching. One second it is serenely quiet. The next second, you want to put your hand over your ears and crouch.

This was the same feeling and experience I had upon awaking well over a year after my injury.

In fact, from March 2010 through my first summer as a brain injury survivor was, by far, the toughest time I have ever lived through. Nothing in my life, no experience I've ever had, would help me in dealing with the reality that unfolded every day.

Mornings, my eyes would open like they have every day of my life. But, just like Hanks' character in Cast Away, my wake-up call was the screaming of tinnitus and other new sounds that are part of the new soundtrack of my life.

My first waking thoughts, my first conscious thoughts, my first awareness of virtually every morning for many months, were of shock and horror.

I would arise to the screaming sounds, making the possibility of going back to sleep not practical. I would think to myself, "Oh my God, I am living with a brain injury", and roll out of bed on unsteady feet as my newfound vertigo made many mornings feel like I was at sea, all in the comfort and familiarity of my own home.

By this time, I had already been diagnosed with both Post Concussive Syndrome and Post Traumatic Stress Disorder. My new normal included the never ending sounds, vertigo, and the very real reality that at any moment in time, I could walk through another amnesia event, and the constant fear of having a seizure became yet another layer of emotional white noise.

At some point in my reading, I stumbled across an interesting statistic. Though I don't recall the source, it was presented that 68% of folks that had what I had, experienced a seizure within the first nine months after the brain trauma. I now lived in the land of the 68 percenters.

Every day, I lived with the reality that there was a 68% chance that I would wake up on the floor, in an ambulance, perhaps in an Emergency Room. Or, perhaps, I wouldn't wake up at all. I am profoundly grateful that this painful chapter is now well in the rearview mirror of my life. One of my new realities is this: I must experience the good and in many cases, the horrific challenges associated with brain injury to grow from this experience.

Very little spiritual growth occurs when life is easy and uneventful. Someone much wiser than me once remarked that pain is the touchstone of all spiritual progress.

I was struggling to pull together pieces of my old life. Trying to get back to work on a full time basis (something I still aspire to do) and hoping that time would ease the pure discomfort of my brain injury. As you've already seen, recovery from a brain injury is like riding on a pendulum.

Sometimes it swings toward a bit of wellness and I deeply embrace that part of the ride. While other times, it swings into complete darkness and despair. When the arc is in that direction, I hold on for dear life. Fortunately, time has shown that while the pendulum of life with MTBI still swings, over time, the arc is less. That does not mean that I have no bad days, I just swing less into the deepest of darkness.

There are two events that best define this particularly dark chapter of my new life.

The first event was terrifying.

Before I get into more detail, I will share that I do at times feel a bit like Superman. There have been so many convoluted and unexpected twists in this journey that there really isn't much that scares me anymore. You come to a point in your stride where you've walked through so much, that the unplanned for, the unexpected, virtually lose their power over you.

I'm not sure whether it's simply a deeper acceptance of the new normal, or if it's more of an "I've come this far and not fallen yet" attitude, but I find myself today not being held hostage by fear. Whatever will come to pass will pass. I can choose to accept this as part of the inherent nature of being human, or I can fight it.

At least for today, I choose acceptance.

The first event is seared so deeply into my memory that it feels like just yesterday, though it was almost a year ago at the time of this writing.

Climbing out of bed to face yet another day, I did what I have been doing most mornings for years. No, it was not a peek out the window, nor was it as mundane as flipping on the news. No, I rolled out of bed and headed for the bathroom.

Passing the vanity mirror on my way to my appointed task, I was caught by complete and unadulterated surprise. The reflection in mirror caught my eye. I paused to look at the reflection and realized that I didn't recognize the face in the mirror.

While my pre-Impact life was about as normal as anyone could hope for, life post-Impact continued its relentless march down Surrealism Avenue. There were so many events, so many incidents and occurrences that I had no prior experience to draw from. No past memories to play connect the dots with; no feeling of déjà vu. So much was new, unfamiliar, uncomfortable and just plain scary.

If I had to guess, I would say that I stood in front of the mirror on that day for a full five minutes or more. My eyes scanned the face looking back. Common sense becomes uncommon sense after a brain injury. I knew it was me.

But I had no idea who "I" was anymore.

I ran my hand across my cheek, looked deeply into unfamiliar eyes, and let confusion wash over me. Until nature called out a bit louder, reminding me why I was there. There is a line in one of my favorite songs that sums it up well.

"Who am I? We both don't know..."

The second event during the Dark Months was actually a significant turning point for me, though I knew it not at the time.

Months earlier, in an effort to make the ongoing and overwhelming chronic headaches a bit more manageable, I was prescribed Amitriptyline. God works in funny ways.

During this dark time on my road to recovery, I experienced a level of despair that was unlike anything I had ever experienced. And why shouldn't I? I was dealing with the most debilitating injury I had ever experienced. Published information from trusted sources said that I would never return to "normal" and the latest round of symptoms from my accident had made the business of daily living hard and uncomfortable.

I wanted out. Stop this ride, let me get off.

And I thought again of suicide.

Not a fun or popular topic to discuss, it is what it is. At one point during this time, I had placed a call to a local Brain Injury Association looking for some information. What should have been a five minute information gathering call went on for close to 30 minutes.

The woman who had taken my call was a volunteer with the organization. In conversation, I asked her if she was a brain injury survivor. Though not a survivor, she had worked for a law firm for many years. She was part of a team that had won a multi-million dollar judgment for a brain injury survivor.

I asked her if that had been the impetus for her commitment to volunteer at the local organization.

Her reply, though well-intentioned was ill-timed.

"Within a couple of weeks of being notified that she was to be the recipient of a multimillion dollar judgment in her favor, she killed herself."

I was stunned on a couple of levels. What did not surprise me were the actions of this fellow sufferer. I understand from an insider's standpoint how traumatizing a brain injury can be. How lonely the road can feel. How overwhelming it can all be.

What stunned me was the fact that she made the decision to share this intimate story with a brain injury survivor. Just imagine if I had cancer, called my local Cancer Association, and was told by the receptionist of people who lost their battle. It's really no different than the call I had. The lyrics were different, but the music was the same.

The second piece that was a shocker was the complete lack of any real compassion. Here was a professional, working for a brain injury association, who shared the tale of the demise of a fellow sufferer with the same tone she would use to recite a shopping list: Devoid of emotion and compassion. Happily, as you will see, there are true and caring compassionate care providers who really understand all of the challenges that survivors face.

Many brain injury sufferers do indeed die from their injuries, just not at the time of impact. Some take months, and even years to succumb to their injuries. Such was the case just presented to me.

And I was on the cusp of calling it quits as well.

And Fate intervened again in the form of an earthborn angel - an angel who saved my life, though she knew it not.

Though my own personal friends list had diminished greatly, I have a very small circle of people who love me unconditionally and who stuck by me through thick and thin. They love me enough to look beyond the brain injury and still see me as a person. They are able to move beyond the discomfort that many feel and though virtually all my relationships have changed form in one way or another, these few people are part of the human network I have come to cherish.

While I skidded along the emotional bottom that threatened to overcome my very desire to live, I had a conversation with a friend over a thousand miles away. At one point, he was one of my customers, but life has a way of taking hold and leading you in directions you don't really plan on.

Over time, Gordon and I become close friends. Phone conversations leaned less to work and more toward life. During this time in my journey, he knew all was not well. Virtually anyone close to me knew this. I had gone from outgoing, gregarious and confident, to sullen, introspective, withdrawn, and yes, suicidal.

And a great secret was revealed.

While on the phone with my long-distance friend, he shared with me something I never knew. His long-term life partner was also a brain injury survivor. Twenty years earlier, she had a traumatic brain injury. For as many years as I knew my long distance friend, I never knew the rest of his story.

I was secretly still holding out hope that I might, just might, mind you, be one of those rare cases of 100% recovery. After a few minutes on the phone, and asking what life was like 20 years after a brain injury, he said quite bluntly, "Why don't you just ask her?" and he put her on the line.

We spoke for thirty minutes or more. She did more speaking, while I hung on every word. Yes, she never got back to her old life completely, but a new life had emerged since her accident, a life very much worth living. She was still a nurse, but worked in a different, more rewarding capacity that would not have come to pass had it not been for her accident. As you'll see shortly, there is so much good that has come out of all of this. We talked very briefly about medications. Meclizine for my vertigo and Amitriptyline for my chronic headaches were discussed.

Her immediate response saved my life, though she may never know it.

"Amitriptyline will make you want to kill yourself."

Eight words delivered with candor from both a nurse as well as a brain injury survivor. No one, not my doctor, not my closest friends, not even Sarah knew the level of desperation I lived in. And here was a voice from someone I've never met; delivering a message from over 1,000 miles away that saved my life.

I never took Amitriptyline again.

Within 48 hours, the urge to end my life ceased abruptly and never returned.

As you know by now, my intent is to not dispense any type of medical advice. I offer what amounts to both a laypersons as well as an insider's view concerning living with a brain injury.

The Amitriptyline was prescribed to me by a neurologist. Never was I warned of side effects. Yes, every medication can have side effects. I'm sure the actual prescription had one of those five page inserts when I picked it up. The lawyers of the world see that that happens.

I am one of the blessed ones. Call it what you will. God? The Spirit of the Universe? Karma? It matters not what you call it. The fact that I was presented with a solution at a time when I could well have been days away from the end of my life is so much more than a coincidence. The timing of her message and the almost immediate cessation of my dark thoughts was the beginning of major change for me. Though life has never gotten back to where I was before my accident, I had new hope that things were going to get better. And they did.

Chapter 12

The Power of Humor

[129]

Coming to grips with life after brain injury takes time; in my case, a long time. Even still, there are days I wake up, open my eyes to a new day, and am confronted by the never ending and often overwhelming ear ringing. And I again experience and relive the shock and disbelief that I am living with a brain injury.

Still, there are other days that I may make it through my first couple of hours and not even think about it. There has not been, however, a day where I don't even think about it. Perhaps that day will come.

In the meantime, I have a life to live. Brain injury or not, the sun will rise and set today, people go to work, they will take care of their children; they suit up and they show up.

To the vast majority of the civilized world, the fact that I live daily with a brain injury does not matter.

But it matters to me.

I have long overcome hardship in life by using humor as a coping tool. Ask anyone over 50 and they will tell you that life passes quickly. Ask anyone over 70 and they will most likely look back on their life and marvel at the speed that it all passes by.

I steadfastly refuse to let my brain injury beat me. A life changed can still be a life worth living. And the pure, unadulterated power of humor has carried me through the darkest of times.

In *The TBI Guide,* Dr. Glen Johnson talks about a commonality among those with a brain injury. Though they may look, sound and in many cases, act the same, almost universally, they remark that they "feel different." In my case, I have an unfamiliar person living in a familiar body. I did not react to situations like "the old David" did. Over time, the process was akin to being introduced to someone you had a nodding familiarity with. Like learning to drive a new car with the controls in unexpected places, I was learning to drive "the new David."

Like an adolescent learning to drive a vehicle with a clutch for the first time, I had innumerable occasions to stall my own personal vehicle; to give it too much gas; to hit the brakes too fast and to want to simply throw my hands up in the air and say "I give up."

It was on one of those days that Sarah and I walked into our local supermarket and I was going on and on about not knowing who I was anymore. So, I decided to start my life all over again with a new name.

"David died the day of the accident," I said to Sarah. "There is no more David."

By now, at over six months since my accident, she was intimately familiar with my struggles and took most of my ranting in stride.

"Who do you want to be?" she asked.

We spent the rest of that shopping trip walking up and down the aisles of our local grocery store deciding who I was going to be moving forward.

"Maybe I'll be Tom, or Bill, or John," doing nothing more than putting together a random list of names. Truth be told, I was tired of being David and it was time for a change.

Never one to be shy, while we paid for our purchases, I asked the cashier who I should be. I let her know I was looking for a new name and a new identity. She took a moment, appeared to be pondering deeply, and said that I would make a good Steve. I thanked her for my newfound identity, grabbed my grocery bags and walked out of the market giggling with Sarah.

You know by now that I am still David. But at that moment in time, I was ready to be just about anyone else. Sarah and I got a big chuckle out of it, but that night she still said "good night David."

My fate was sealed.

This journey has taken so many odd and unexpected twists and turns. While many are bitter and painful, others can be at times downright comical. Let's talk about Aphasia, shall we?

By definition, Aphasia is *"the partial or total loss of the ability to articulate ideas or comprehend spoken or written language, resulting from damage to the brain caused by injury."*

In simple terms, I was left with a speech disorder after my accident. There is an irony in all of this. I am, by nature, a consummate communicator. My written work has been published nationally on several occasions. Over the span of the last 20+ years, I have spoken to groups on a wide range of topics and have been told repeatedly that I've been given the gift of being able to articulate various subjects and concepts with ease.

Wasn't I surprised 3-4 months after my accident, when I started to lose the ability to speak? It started with the gradual misplacement of words.

"Sarah, can you stop by the stone on the way home from work?" I would ask innocently.

"Do you mean the store?"

Over a window of time lasting only a few weeks, my ability to get more than a couple of sentences out without misspeaking, all but fell by the wayside. Keep in mind that this happened months after my accident.

I still wrestle with speech challenges. Though not noticeable to most, I speak more slowly than I ever have. Lost is the ability to just talk. I must, at a conscious level, think about the exact words I want to say and then follow my thoughts with the act of speaking. It's become a bit of a one-two Waltz to communicate. But, though I must go through this sometimes tedious process to speak, it has gotten easier Most who know me will never notice.

And I laugh. More deeply, my from my soul, than I ever have.

A recent visit to one of my doctors found me telling her I was "unable to put two sandwiches together anymore." My intent was to share that two *sentences* together were a challenge. We sat in her office and laughed.

A bit later, I'll get into what are called "adaptive strategies." These are nothing more than new ways to do what used to come naturally. As memory problems remain problematic to this day and, the very nature of my life demands attention to detail and considerable recall, my propensity to forget quickly became a major source of angst and frustration.

In what amounted to a moment of brilliance, I decided to use yellow sticky notes to remember things. Being one who has embraced technology, I opted not for the old peel away paper sticky notes. No, I was smarter than that, or so I thought.

As my day revolves largely around working in my office, I chose the more 21st century approach - digital sticky notes. Every time something that I deemed likely to forget would cross my mind, I would add a new sticky note to my desktop.

On the surface, one would think this to be an effective adaptive strategy. But there was one small flaw in the model. Something I never would have expected.

A month after I decided to use the digital sticky method of recalling day-to-day facts, I noticed something on my monitor. It was yellow and familiar. Had it been tactile, it would have been covered with dust.

What was it? It was my unread pile of digital reminders. By this time, they went back weeks and the information I thought so critical to remember was now unimportant and in the past.

I laughed; so much for that adaptive strategy! It did, however, prompt me to put a new note on top of my pile of sticky notes. My first note, almost in a bit of self-effacing jest said, "Remember to read your sticky notes!"

The list of unexpected quirks seems at times to be never ending. I have learned to laugh at challenges that might make others cry. And why shouldn't I? Looking at all that has happened since my accident can be bittersweet indeed. While so much has been lost, there can be no doubt that my Fate could have been so vastly different than it is. The very fact that I am able to put together reasonably cohesive thoughts in an order that has some semblance of sense is tangible proof that there really is some gray matter left.

Long a fan of cartoon characters, there are times I feel like I have crossed the line into a surrealistic state where most anything is possible. At some point during that first year, at a time I am unable to recall, the realization that my vision was not as it was, was becoming increasingly clear. A visit to my local optometrist disclosed something a bit startling. Gone was much of my ability for my eyes to track distant objects in unison. What exactly does that mean in layman's terms? Simply put, I was knocked slightly cross-eyed from my accident. Not many people have noticed it. There are many times, especially when I am overtired, where my vision simply doubles up. Try as I might, I simply can't straighten out my eyes.

I allow myself the luxury of laughing at it. In a quirky kind of way, it is rather humorous - to be hit hard enough to have my eyes crossed. Perhaps you don't see the humor in it. But for a moment, envision a cartoon character on a Saturday morning kids show get hit with a frying pan. You watch the faux birdies chirping in circles around his head as he swaggers to and fro, eyes crossed. You've no doubt seen the visual. I live it. No birdies, mind you. Not a frying pan in sight, thankfully. But a goofy grin and eyes cast asunder. Yes. That's me.

Brain injury is a wild and wooly West of all that can happen to someone. Yes, it's baffling. Yes, it's funny at times - in a quirky kind of way.

Chapter 13

An Unexpected Revelation

So much of my life has taken on an *Alice in Wonderland* feel that almost nothing is beholden of the power to surprise me anymore. Worth noting is that I said *almost* nothing.

I am a man of Faith. Not the Sunday, church-going kind of faith. Though I have been exposed to a myriad of religions, I call none my own. My birth certificate states that I am a Protestant by baptism. My secondary education was at a Catholic school. Over the years, I've read books on topics ranging from Buddhism to Paganism. My neighborhood at times sees small bands of Mormons or Jehovah's Witnesses out proselytizing their respective causes.

Never one to have a harsh word, I've engaged more than just a few of these folks in spirited, well-intentioned debate.

My own belief set is more of a practical belief set. Born of faith, fueled by science, and crowned with a child-like belief in the Goodness of the Universe, I can say from the depths of my being that there is

Something out there beyond human comprehension that watches over us all.

Looking at the world purely through the eyes of science, ponder this: as you read these words, you are on a ball of rock hurdling through space at over 66,000 miles an hour. Look down at your feet for a moment. Only a few miles beneath you is a core of molten lava that has been churning for millions of years.

Look above you. A few miles up, all air is gone, the temperature falls to absolute zero and life as we know it cannot be sustained.

Yet, amid this chaos above and below us, we live; we thrive. If our planet were a mere few thousand miles closer to the Sun, our planet would be too warm to support life. Move us a few thousand miles in the other direction, and the Earth is too cold to support life as we know it.

Yet here we are. In the celestial "sweet spot", where life not only has come to pass, but where it flourishes with almost reckless abandon.

Sure, some may call this a coincidence of grandiose proportion. But, not me. The more learned men and woman force science to disclose her secrets to humanity, the more far-fetched the very thought that this may all be by chance.

Coincidence is a funny thing. By definition, coincidence is "the occurrence of events remarkable either for being simultaneous or for apparently being connected."

I think of coincidence as being something a bit different. Coincidence to me is a glimpse behind the curtain: A tangible moment in time where a life experience reveals to us that a deeper realm, far greater than we are able to perceive at a conscious level, is part of the veritable fabric of our existence.

As 2011 continued to pass, life took on a bit of a new and familiar rhythm. My "new normal" was becoming familiar. Not always comfortable and not always easy, it was slowly and over time becoming a bit easier. Gone were the days I could pound out a full day of work Gone were the days when I could sit in silence- even for a moment. Gone was the innocence of life before brain injury.

But I was evolving. Changing, learning, and living.

My old routines were replaced by new ones. Daily, I would work in front of my PC diligently until 2:00 PM, then crash with a level of mental exhaustion so overwhelming, I was unable to even find familiar keys on my keyboard.

Being one of the lucky brain injury survivors, my mental exhaustion did not transcend into my physical realm. By 2:30 PM most days, I would be back in Spandex and back on my bike for my daily 30+ mile bike ride, my daily cardio forcing highly oxygenated blood through my still healing brain.

And monthly, I would attend my MTBI Support Group. It was at one of these get-togethers that the Universe revealed yet another "coincidence."

Every few months, our regular monthly meeting would open to the family and friends of the regular attendees. It remains a great way for the husbands, wives, partners, mothers, and fathers, anyone whose life is touched by a TBI, to come together.

A fellow brain injury survivor had her husband by her side. Though I looked familiar to him, he had no element of familiarity to me at all. Why should he? The only time we had met was when I was being strapped onto a gurney to be taken to our local trauma center the day of my accident.

Stranger than fiction, the husband of one of the regular members of my support group was one of the local police officers on-scene the day of my accident. To some who calculate odds, they might be inclined to say it's a 1 in 1,000 chance, but it can happen.

Not me. I call it a 100% chance. We met again because we were supposed to. And the conversation that ensued was nothing short of one of the grandest revelations of my life.

The conversation unfolded, in all places, in the lobby of a local cinema where our brain injury support group had its first field trip as a group. The 2012 release of The Vow, a movie whose main plot was centered on a brain injury survivor seemed to be a good choice for our first ever group outing.

Husbands, wives and family members were all invited. Tears and popcorn flowed freely as we all watched characters on the big screen who had life challenges similar to our own. We laughed, we cried, and shared a time none of us would have envisioned even a few short years ago.

Lingering in the lobby after the movie, no one seemed too rushed to end our get together. Small groups of two and three broke out and conversations unfolded.

I found myself in the company of the husband of one of our group members. I had known for a couple of months that he was on-scene immediately after my accident as one of the responding first officers that had been dispatched. Yet this was the first time I had the opportunity to speak with him.

His first comment to me opened up an amazing insight as to exactly what happened the day I was hit.

"I'm glad you are alive."

Emotions abounded and tears crept close to the surface. Here was my chance to ask questions that would help me to perhaps understand better the events of that fated day. There were still so many questions I had, so many blank spots, so much I longed to understand.

And the kind hand of Fate had unexpectedly put the answers I was seeking directly in front of me.

Unasked for. Unexpected. Unbidden.

Afraid of what I might hear, my first question was one of curiosity. "What kind of shape was the car that hit me in?"

His reply was so out of the realm of anything I expected to hear, yet explained so much. One of the most poignant memories I have of the accident scene was of the passer-by who was unable to stop weeping. Hand covering her mouth, she wept. I lay there, body broken and mind numbed on Main Street, unable to look away from this complete stranger watching me while she cried.

It was a defining moment at the accident scene as it was the face of this unwitting fellow member of our human family that made me think that I may not live to see another sunrise.

Laying there on Main Street, I knew that I was hurt, and hurt badly. But until the weeping stranger entered my field of vision, I had fully expected to brush it off, maybe deal with a couple of scrapes and bruises, and jump back into my life in no time.

As you've read already, my default setting is, and remains, one of optimism under most any and all circumstances.

The Officer went on to describe in exquisite detail exactly what he saw and what he experienced.

"The entire front end of the car that hit you was pushed in," he began. "But it was the windshield that took most of the impact. The whole windshield was pushed into the front seat of the car."

"Had anyone been a passenger in the car, he would have been seriously injured because the windshield was in the front seat."

"Though the entire windshield was pushed in, perhaps four feet of it," he continued, "the most damage was in front of the passenger's seat where your head literally went through the windshield leaving a hole where your helmet was."

I was stunned. Yes, I knew that the scene was chaotic. The sheer number of first responders let me know that. But the degree of damage to the vehicle left me shocked. Had I found myself in the shoes of virtually anyone on scene, eyes drifting from the crumbled body on the pavement and back to the carnage that was formerly a drivable vehicle, I probably would have wondered as well if the cyclist was going to survive.

And yes, tears would have been flowing down my face as well.

My understanding of why some of the events that came to pass crystallized with clarity previously unknown.

The fear and mortal concern I saw in the eyes of those attending to me suddenly made sense. The urgency of the screams to "call 9-1-1" made sense. The fact that my local police department sent an officer across state lines to the trauma center to get a statement from me now made sense. My survival was not guaranteed.

I now understood why Sarah spent days after the accident pulling glass out of my scalp with tweezers. And I now knew why my helmet was full of small sections of hair that were sheared off my head by the very force of the accident.

Prior to this conversation, if you had asked me about damage to the vehicle that hit me, I most likely would have said that it had sustained not much more than a cracked windshield and a possible dent or two.

Yet right in front of me stood a man telling me about an accident far grander, far more intense and far more serious that I ever imagined.

We talked for a few more minutes about other events that came to pass that day. None, however, were as revealing as the first-hand description of what passed that day.

How did it feel, hearing such descriptive details about an event that has forever changed me?

Truth be told, it was freeing. Unanswered questions were no more and I was left feeling profoundly grateful. Grateful that Fate brought us together and grateful that the meeting was well after the one-year anniversary of my accident. I had healed enough by this time to understand the full implications of what unfolded at the accident scene and, I was far enough along my new road to not let the new details completely overwhelm me.

Who knows how I would have reacted to his story had it been revealed to me in the first few months after the accident? Thankfully, that was not the case. By the time the full tale was revealed, I was already well underway in the process of embracing my new life.

Chapter 14

Adapt and Thrive

As my first year as a brain injury survivor continued to pass, it became very clear that my old way of living, though effective for close to half a century, would need a complete overhaul.

Ask most any brain injury survivor which three words fully describe the frustration of living with a brain injury, and you'll most likely hear, "You look normal."

Like so many others, my physical injuries healed as they should have. Broken bones knit and healed, bruises turned from black to green to yellow and faded slowly with the passage of time. The hair that was shorn from my head from the violent and abrupt force of impact grew back over time.

But my brain became unreliable for many of my day-to-day tasks. The ability to effectively judge the passage of time eludes me to this day. Life events are either in the moment, in the future, or in the past. Once an event comes to pass, I am hard pressed to tell you whether it occurred last week or a year ago.

Though I do my best to smile at this oddity, it can be embarrassing at times.

As you've read already, my ability to feel cold has left the building. I have had to weave new and unexpected compensatory strategies into my life.

Over time, these new coping mechanisms are becoming more second nature than they were in the beginning. So much of moving forward simply feels like buying time: finding ways to move forward, to stay busy, and to not think about the degree to which I was injured.

I'll be devoting quite a bit of time on this as the development of new coping skills has been one of the largest pieces of the puzzle that has fallen into place with all that involves living with a brain injury. By focusing on living my life as best I can, it's inevitable that time will pass and that I will, however haltingly, move forward.

And time has proven this to be true.

There have been so many timelines for my recovery that have been bantered about by medical professionals. The first neurologist I saw estimated that I would be back at 100% within six months. A few months later, he changed his projection to 12-18 months. At the time of our last visit, he said it could be five years or more. At one year after my accident, a leading area neurologist let me know that I was "permanently disabled." This troubling diagnosis came at the one year anniversary of my accident. You'll read more about that later.

Recovery timelines are very much moving targets in respect to brain injury.

In *My Stroke of Insight*, Dr. Jill Bolte Taylor speaks of measurable gains up to eight years after a brain injury. Spend just a short time researching brain injury recovery times and you'll see a vast gulf between the extremes.

Time has shown me that my brain will recover at its own pace. Early on, I put too much emphasis on trying to get back to "normal." Placing a huge amount of pressure on myself, pressure that lead to undue stress, sleepless nights and constant fear, I worried when I marched by each milestone on my journey.

At six months, the degree to which I was hurt was beginning to become clear. By one year, my hopes of overcoming brain injury started to evaporate.

Today I try to remind myself that there really is no timeline. Recovery will be life-long and it's really my attitude and not the calendar that matters.

There has been a common misconception that most recovery occurs within the first year after a brain injury. I've read this fact online on many sites that claim to offer clinical information. In fact, I have been told this very fact by members of the medical community.

I deem the presentation of this type of timeline to be a real disservice to those who have suffered a brain injury. From the standpoint of a survivor, to be told that at the one year mark "you'll be as good as you'll get" can become an impassable barrier to moving forward.

In my own case, some of my biggest gains were close to the 18 month mark. In fact, it was at 18 months that I started what I call the process of "waking up."

Though challenges still presented, it was at the year and a half point that I knew I was going to be OK.

An attendee at my monthly MTBI support group shared that year three was her breakthrough year. It bears restating that I present a laypersons point of view about recovery. Everyone has their own journey. My experience is just that - It is what I have walked though. Yours, or that of someone you love, will be different.

The point is this: If you've been told that you've reached the point where there will be no further gains, honor the recovery process and don't give up hope. I fully expect to be recovering for the rest of my life. But when you really think about it, aren't we all recovering from something?

As my march toward wellness continues, there are other adaptive strategies that have made my life infinitely more manageable. While some are more common sense strategies, others are a bit more non-mainstream.

In sharing with other survivors, time management seems to be an almost universal challenge. By time management, I am not referencing the Corporate America, *I have too much to do and not enough time to do it*, type of time management challenges.

Not even close. Effective time management in my case is oddly much simpler than that. For many months after my accident, I experienced grand frustration by not knowing what day of the week it was. In fact, I was hard pressed to tell you the month at any given time…the year? Don't even ask.

There is a bit of a comical element to that as well. Seasons in the Northeast have, for most of my lifetime, been rather predictable. Flowers bloom in the spring. Days get longer and lawns need mowing in the summer. Trees turn color and days get shorter in the fall.

And in the winter, it snows.

Most winters, that is. In the winter that followed my one year accident anniversary, we had a virtually snowless winter here in New England. It was a bit bittersweet. Never one to enjoy clearing the driveway of snow, I really did enjoy a winter where local snow shovels did nothing more than gather dust.

But an unexpected challenge arose. Looking out my window, the landscape never changed. For close to five months, trees remained barren, leaves littered brown lawns, and no snow came. I was hard pressed to tell you whether it was October or March.

It was in a fit of frustration that Sarah again came to my rescue. This time, salvation came in the form of a watch. With clear placement on the main watch face, I was able to read the day of the week, the month and even the year.

While this may sound like a small challenge to many, my inability to remember the day and month was a constant source of frustration and more than an occasional source of embarrassment.

A multi-function watch with an affordable price tag virtually eliminated this source of anxiety from my life. I still find myself glancing at my watch 15-20 times a day to get a bit of a spot check as to where I am in the chronological scheme of things. Such a small cost in relation to the quality of life it helped me to achieve.

Most all of my compensatory strategies have come to me like this. Not by reading about them in a book, or hearing about them. Most start with the awareness that there is some type of deficiency. From that awareness, initial frustrations abounded as I tried to use my old methodology of coping, only to find it lacking. It is out of that frustration that my quest for a solution to a specific problem begins.

Let's talk about memory for a while, shall we?

Memory challenges are almost universal among brain injury survivors. From my online research and learning sessions to time spent with others whose fates mirror my own, I hear tales of memory challenges repeated with an uncanny frequency.

As you read about in my snow globe analogy, the recall of pre-injury memories remains largely untainted. In fact, many of my own life memories that were laid down before my accident have an unexpected and crystalline clarity.

Recently, a childhood friend tracked me down on Facebook. We attended fifth grade together. To add the benefit of a bit of timeline framework to this, it had been over 39 years since we sat side-by-side in a fifth grade classroom.

[157]

Suffice to say, more than just a little life passes by in 39 years. Yet the shocker was my recall of a specific day back in the early 1970's as we walked home from elementary school. My recall of the route we took, even a few snippets of the conversation came flooding back. Here I was, on the north side of 50 years old, recalling a childhood conversation.

The power of the human brain to store information is absolutely mind-boggling. Long before my accident, these specific memories were stored somewhere in my brain, yet my ability to recall them, to access the specific files that contained these memories, was lost.

It is experiences like these that, oddly enough, have offered me the greatest hope. My brain has shown, by living example, that this data, this information, has not been lost. Rather, as time continues to show, my ability to access older memories has indeed been profoundly enhanced by my accident.

The biggest challenge, by far, remains my ability to access memories that were created after my accident. Looking back over the first year of my post-accident life, it is painfully clear that for a lot of the year, my lights were indeed on, though no one was home.

Larger blocks of time from that first year are essentially gone. If those memories have been somehow archived in my brain to be accessed later, only time will tell.

As the months passed in my post-impact life, the consequences of my memory loss became painfully clear.

Though only able to work on a part-time basis, I struggled valiantly to regain control of my business. As most of my business is built on relationships, many of them long-term by the time my accident had occurred, I had a number of clients who, upon being offered more details about what had befallen me, were more than willing to wait it out.

They had the experience of working with me prior to my injury and knew from real-world experience what I was like when I was on top of my game. To this day, I am both humbled and profoundly grateful for the core clients I have come to know and love over the years that "waited it out."

The real challenge on a professional level was those clients who became part of my business family only after my accident. They had not the experience of working with me at my prime and were only able to gauge what I was capable of based on my post-impact level of professional performance.

As one who has an unwavering commitment to a professional standard far above the norm, both seeing how I fell short of my expectations daily and to hear new clients speak openly about my inability to meet commitments were perhaps one of the low points in my first year.

Many depended upon me before my accident. Though Sarah and I are technically a two income family, both incomes are required to keep the gears of our lives turning. To have either of us out of work for any type of extended time means hardship. I was back at my desk within a week after my accident more out of fear than any real desire to be working. Not working has never been an option.

As time passed, there were certain parts of my work-a-day life that were clearly those causing the most problems. For example: setting up a conference call with a new client only to remember the scheduled call a day after the appointment is really not conducive to building a long lasting business relationship.

Letting a client know that a project would be completed within a week, only to get a call two weeks later by a client looking for an update is not the way to grow a business. From a self-worth and esteem standpoint, these experiences were humiliating, humbling and the cause of immense concern.

That still, small voice that we all have constantly whispered negativity to me. "David, you've lost your edge and it's never coming back," was part of my new daily internal monologue. "Not only will it never get better, it may likely get worse." The list goes on. Like a narrator offering an internal commentary on all my shortcomings, I sat in my own private screening room and wondered if life as I knew it was ever going to be the same.

Then it hit me: the integrity of my work was untainted! A significant part of my job involves the creation of content for clients. Whether text or graphics, I have long created content viewed very favorably by my clients. The challenges I faced were not the result of inferior work. Rather, almost across the board, my challenges involved time management.

At one point along the way, my neurologist suggested that I do as many "outside of the brain" tasks as possible. He went on to suggest that by removing these tasks from my brain I would free up more of my internal system resources.

Earlier I shared with you the challenge of my sticky notes; dozens of reminders set for everything from time to take breaks to project deadlines. I still smile at the fact that most all of my sticky notes were never read and that I continued to make notes then promptly forget about them.

It became clear that there needed to be another attempt at finding a way to schedule tasks. There is an old adage that says, *"If you keep doing what you are doing, you'll keep getting what you are getting."* What I was doing needed to be changed if I was to find a way to move forward professionally.

And there is a distinct link to my own sense of self that comes from my work. No, I am not my job, but I am forever linked to what I do. This is probably more so with folks like me who are self-employed, as there really Is no time clock to punch at 5:00 PM and simply call it a day.

I need to share as well that my compensatory strategies are my own. I have met others whose strategies are far different than mine and work very well. The important point for me was to simply keep trying and to find a way to the other side of the barriers that my brain injury placed in front of me. For once, my stubbornness was about to pay off.

The process started with my need to have all my information at my fingertips. Project deadlines, scheduled appointments, scheduled calls with clients, all of this needed to be within easy reach.

Initially I gave thought to an online calendar of sorts. A web-based extension of my own memory where I could post the type of details that would help my life run more smoothly. After test-driving a couple of web-based services, I settled into a comfortable routine of using Google calendar. It quickly became apparent that it fit me like a glove. It was intuitive for me to use. Tasks like phone calls and customer appointments were quickly added to my calendar.

The results were nothing short of life changing. It took a couple of weeks to get into the habit of checking my calendar every morning to see what the day ahead was going to hold. Happily, that is now a habit for me.

I aim for progress and not perfection as I journey in my recovery. Yes, there is still a very infrequent missed call. But the number of missed calls and appointments has dropped by over 95%. My ability to recall specific appointments may or may not ever come back, but my ability to recall the two-part process of using a calendar works very nicely.

First I am sure to add what needs my attention to my calendar. Next up, I now habitually check it. Though someone without a brain injury may think this to be just common sense, it was not for me. For years, I was able to hold memories in my mind and juggle a very complex schedule without the need for this type of ongoing documentation.

Whether or not that ever comes back to me no longer matters. My new methodology for "out of the brain" recall works just fine.

The real "win" here is that my confidence is back; my esteem is no longer rocked when an important date is missed, and life between my ears is dramatically less stressful. The issue was identified, a new strategy was developed and implemented, and I was free to move forward to work on finding a way to make the next piece of the puzzle fit.

My next strategy may not really be so much compensatory, but more so a coping strategy.

As you've read on a couple of occasions, my ability to experience true silence has been robbed from me by my accident. Thrust into the new and uncomfortable world of tinnitus, I live with perpetual ear ringing. Not intermittent in nature, from the moment my eyes open to greet a new day until I lean over to kiss Sarah goodnight, my ears ring.

Not a soft chime or easy-listening type of ringing. No, this is a veritable freight train of sound that is with me every waking minute of every day. Akin to what I envision Chinese water torture must feel like, my attitude swings from resigned acceptance to an overwhelming desire to rip my ears off my head.

My tinnitus continues, to this day, to be one of the lasting effects of my brain injury that I would do just about anything to correct.

During the latter part of the first year of my post-impact life, I set up an appointment to see a local audiologist. I had reached a point of complete and utter frustration. For months, I simply let time pass, hoping against hope that it would correct itself.

Heading into the audiologist's office that morning for testing, I held out hope that there may be something to be done to lift this curse from me. A bit of online reading showed nothing promising, yet the doctor was quite interested in seeing me.

On a bit of a side note here, I work very hard at not being negative. Negativity is a barrier to forward progress and recovery. It robs me of vital strength and resources I need to move closer to wellness. But there have been some experiences along the way that simply befuddle me.

After spending close to an hour with an office assistant going through diagnostics of all sorts, it was time to have a sit-down with the doctor to go over my next steps. What happened over the course of the next 15 minutes left me stunned and disheartened.

He quite kindly went over the results of my hearing tests and was pleased with the overall test results. So far, so good. He then "confirmed" my tinnitus and said quite bluntly that there was nothing that could be done; that there was no effective treatment.

He went on to paint a picture of many people so desperate that they would do almost anything to silence the ringing. This level of desperation, he continued, spawned the creation of an entire scam industry intended to prey upon this level of desperation. He closed our session with the comment that tinnitus, while perceived as an ear problem, does not actually originate in the ear. It is more aptly described as a neurological issue.

And in the wink of an eye, more hope was lost. The most natural question to ask would be why I was not told when the office was first called that it was untreatable. Sarah and I walked out of his office, with hundreds of dollars of additional medical debt that could have been avoided.

And the ringing continued on.

Compensatory strategies have consistently come to me at low points along this new road I am walking. From memory lapses forcing "out of the brain" solutions to the constant internal choir between my ears, I have used pain, discomfort and frustration as springboards to move me forward. Realistically, what other choice is there?

The night-time ringing was made more tolerable by our bedside white noise machine. Sarah and I still travel several times a year and I marvel at her ability to move forward with life at a pace and grace that I envy. While away, as she unpacks an overnight bag, out comes the white noise machine from our bedside. It's traveled more than many people I know and has seen the likes of several states as well as a trip or two to Walt Disney World!

But how was I to make daily life easier? If the ringing was not going away, how could I coexist with it?

The night time challenges were not the issue. My biggest challenge was the 40+ hours I spend at my desk. As my work requires intense focus, soft music in the background, while suitable for some, was not going to work. It would leave me distracted, unproductive and frustrated. As I wrestle with a new level of A.D.D. since impact, music while I worked was tantamount to a recipe for disaster.

Sometime solutions are so simple, so blatant, that you wonder how they were missed. Such was the solving of my daytime dilemma.

Sitting on my desk now is a five gallon fish tank. Yes, my ever-present new friends are nice, but they are secondary. (Just don't tell them.) The real benefit here is the soft hum of the filter. A period of trial and error ensued after the tank made its way to my desktop, as the "whisper quiet" filters were too quiet. A small aerator in the tank, emitting a constant stream of bubbles to entertain my aquatic friends, kicked up the volume just enough to drown out some of the ringing.

An investment of less than fifty dollars continues to this day to pay dividends toward my peace of mind and my sanity.

Rather than look at the enormity of living with overwhelming tinnitus every day, it has helped me to compartmentalize my life. It's always easier to take small bites out of an apple than to eat it all in one bite. My daytimes became immensely easier and my night times did so as well - All of this with no real reduction in the level of my ringing, but by implementing strategies to make life easier.

Solutions are funny as once you find something that works you want to run with it. As I start most mornings with a quiet period of reading a daily meditation book and reflecting on what the day may hold, it became my habit to do this by our backyard fishpond. The addition of a small backyard waterfall quickly solved the challenge of my quiet time not really being quiet at all.

As you can see, so much of rebuilding life after brain injury goes well beyond trying to get as healthy as possible. Rather, it is almost a game to identity specific challenges and then work toward creating solutions that help.

Does it really work? I can answer in a heartbeat that yes, these changes have made my life significantly more comfortable. As new challenges arise, I no longer get as discouraged. You see, I now have a history of implementing new methodologies that work. As brain injury is a "two steps forward, one step back" condition, when the back-stepping occurs, I try to do my best to view it as an opportunity to develop a new skill.

This is much harder than it sounds, but the rewards are immeasurable.

By this time, I thought I had a good handle on where I was along my new road. What my next round of testing would reveal was nothing short of shocking.

Chapter 15

Permanently Disabled?

I almost drank the Kool-Aid. Over and over I read that most recovery from a brain injury happens within the first year. From multiple websites to information passed on to me directly by well intentioned doctors, the One Year threshold was supposed to be statistically significant.

Being told that any gains after the one year mark would be minor at best, the one year anniversary of my accident approached and I knew with every fiber of my being that I still had very big life challenges related to my brain injury. My state of mind could best be called despair.

Based on what I was told and what I had read, I hit a low point of resignation that the rest of my life would be defined by near constant vertigo; that I would never know silence as the tinnitus was still in full swing, and any hopes of having a functioning memory were evaporating like a summer rain.

The state I was in was to be my destiny. Sure, I might get a bit better, but not measurably so. My fate was sealed; my destiny determined. I was to relegate myself to a life abounding with challenges and minimal relief.

Or so I thought.

As noted earlier, I in no way present myself as any type of medical authority on brain injury. I'm a pretty average guy who took a tough hit to the head. I am also a writer; hence this book.

But I do have a very unique insight into the realm of brain injury that only comes from living it. If you add together every bit of knowledge I've gleaned from the books I read, the websites I've poured through, the doctors I've talked to, the summation of all of that "outside information" is only a speck of dust compared to what I've learned firsthand by actually living daily with a brain injury.

One of the great revelations in all of this is that no two paths are alike. My brain, unlike any other part of me that might, over the course of my lifetime been injured, takes its own time to recover. Its timeline is its own.

My greatest single period of recovery thus far was at the fifteen to sixteen month point after my accident. At that point, I walked through a period of recovery that was both unexpected and profoundly life-changing. For the first time since my accident, I have moments - moments mind you - of life that was close to normal. I had glimpses of my pre-accident self. It was akin to being reacquainted with an old friend.

No, there was not the absence of all challenges. But it was like the volume was turned down on many of my most glaring symptoms.

If you are reading this and are a brain injury survivor who has been told you are as good as you'll get, I implore you to not pay attention to what you were told. I am glad I chose not to accept what I was told and continued my aggressive road to recovery well beyond the one year point.

At one of my monthly brain injury support group meetings, a member shared that year three was her year of the most gains.

Yes, every journey is different. My experience is part of my own personal journey, and you have your own path to walk. But pay limited attention to those who share information that may hold you back.

As year one wound down, it was time to go on a fact finding mission. I was starting to make slow progress forward and, it was time to get a real feel of the degree that my brain was damaged. It was time for an Independent Medical Examination in the form of exhaustive neuropsychological testing.

Those who know me best know that I am an optimist to the core. In fact, this is yet another reason to be profoundly grateful as I retained this attribute even after my accident. I simply refuse to let a life event, no matter how challenging, change how I feel about the inherent goodness of life.

When it was time to find a neuropsychologist, I had 100% free reign over who I was going to choose. As the insurance company of the young man who hit me walked away from any responsibility of covering my ongoing medical debt, and my own health insurance coverage was a very high deductible catastrophic health plan, I had complete freedom to choose a doctor based on reputation and proficiency alone.

There were no concerns about an in-network doctor, an out of network doctor, a participating doctor and the like. Here is a classic case of what may be perceived by many as a negative (my lack of meaningful health insurance) actually being a blessing.

By this time, I was on a first name basis with many brain injury professionals in my local area. It only took a few days of asking around to find a well-respected neuropsychologist to see.

Overall, the purpose of the neuropsychological testing was to take what amounts to a bit of a brain inventory. The extensive and exhausting testing would reveal in stark detail where my mental and cognitive abilities had been compromised.

As I was still in the mindset that I was about as good as I was going to get, I wanted to use this detailed and specific information to help best formulate a plan to live out my life. To see where I was lacking and to perhaps fine tune my coping and compensatory strategies to best help me move forward.

The actual testing took place over three sessions; close to six hours of testing that was nothing short of grueling.

Truth be told, I have nothing but high regard for the doctor who conducted the testing. Having had decades of experience in working with the brain injured, he laid the groundwork for what was to happen at my first visit.

"We are going to find out exactly what has been compromised. With this information, I can then make recommendations custom tailored to your results, to formulate coping skills to help you," he quite confidently stated during our first visit.

I found his candor refreshing and his focus on developing a personal plan based on his findings to be in alignment with where I wanted to go in the next chapter of my recovery.

There really is no need to get into the specifics of the testing and the testing mechanisms as the meaningful information was to be presented at the conclusion of the testing.

From the get-go, I let the doctor know that I wanted Sarah to be there for what I called The Great Reveal. Not one to trust my compromised memory, I wanted another set of ears and eyes there as we went over what the testing revealed. I knew as well that Sarah would have questions that I may not think to ask. We have been a team through all of this. Her presence at The Great Reveal was a requisite.

By the time the testing was completed and the results compiled, it was early 2012. Keep in mind that I was hit in late 2010. Brain injury recovery timelines are nothing short of patience teachers.

Sarah and I arrived at his office and were told in advance that The Great Reveal would take upwards of an hour.

I was scared.

Terrified, in fact. Like a condemned man going off to meet the executioner, I was expecting to hear how damaged I was and how improbable it would be that I would ever recover.

By now, you are probably thinking that the results were not as dramatic as I am making them out to be, that I was extreme in what my expectations were. That perhaps, I would bc told some very good news.

Oh, how I wish that was to be, but such was not the case at all.

The test results were broken down in segments. There were two areas that deeply concerned the doctor.

In one section, called "Complex Problem Solving," I was in the bottom 5th percentile. The test was scaled to ensure my results matched both my gender and my age group. Simply put, 95% of people my age had problem solving skills that exceeded my ability. I tested out at close to the bottom of the barrel.

The next stunning revelation involved verbal recall. I had known for a long time that I had trouble following conversations since my accident. Sarah and I went, almost weekly, to the movies on our Thursday night date nights and I had long known that following a plotline while watching a movie on the big screen in my new post-impact world was next to impossible.

"David, your verbal recall skills are also in the bottom 5 percentile," the doctor shared.

I was able to suit up and show up, have engaging conversations and, by all appearances, look like there was someone home and that my lights were on.

But appearances can be so deceiving!

By the time most conversations ended, I had almost no recall as to what was discussed.

Like looking back and being able to play connect-the-dots, my lack of any meaningful and real ability to recall verbal dialogue more than explained a few of my challenges. Sarah had said repeatedly over the previous year that I developed a propensity to ask the same question over and over. My lack of ability to recall conversation may not have made this any easier for her, but it did make it understandable.

And then the hammer fell.

"David, you are permanently disabled and any further recovery will most likely be minimal at best."

We sat there in stunned silence. What was left of my mind raced, only to become lost in the full implication of this stunning news.

Here sat a well-schooled, seasoned and trusted doctor who handed me a completely unacceptable sentence

I was only paying half-attention as he continued on about whether I, as a disabled person, would like information about how to apply for government disability benefits.

Me? Permanently disabled? Sorry, Doc, you must have me confused with someone else. In the last year, I continued, however haltingly, to run my business, to live my life, and Sarah and I travelled on occasion. Jeepers, I had even bought a new car a few months earlier.

Does this sound like someone who is permanently disabled?

Yet in my heart, I knew there was an element of truth to what he shared. I had gone to him on a fact-finding mission. And facts I had. The biggest question was this: exactly what was I going to do with this newfound information?

And now date night challenges became clearer.

For a decade or more, Sarah and I have set aside Thursday nights for what we fondly call Date Night. It is our one night a week to get away, just the two of us. We recharge and reconnect without distractions.

Some date nights we take the twenty-five minute ride to the Atlantic coast as there is something cathartic about just being close to the Sea. Heading to a local seaside community near us, a stop for fried dough is sometimes the order of the night. Other times, it's nothing more than the drive to the beach and a walk along the shore holding hands.

But more often than not, date night consists of dinner and a movie. My definition of heaven on Earth is pretty simple. A nice meal, tickets for two at our local cinema, a bit of popcorn and some M&M's. Add Sarah's hand in mine and it ready doesn't get much better.

It became clear in early 2011 that something had changed. The dinner and social part of date night remained largely unchanged. Thank God for small miracles. The actual movie part, however, was vastly different.

We have a long-standing tradition of not supporting violent movies. Though the decision of two movie-goers in New Hampshire will most likely have minimal impact on the movie choices that Hollywood opts for, our passive non-support of violence is simply the way we choose to live our lives. The world has enough terror and scariness in it already without having to pay hard earned money to help propagate it.

Though we were able to select which movies we supported, there was no way to prevent exposure to the movie trailers that were created to entice folks to future shows. As my post-traumatic stress disorder was in high gear, I would shield my eyes or look away as bombs dropped, snipers shot, fireballs exploded, men, women and in some cases children screamed in the type of realism that Hollywood is known for. I would tremble and quake in my padded movie chair awaiting the start of our evening movie.

On several occasions over the course of my first year of post-impact life, I came precariously close to walking out of our local theater. The only thing holding me to my seat was the ever present drone of "I'm not going to let this beat me..." as I forced this thought into an endless loop until the trailers ended. How many times I sat there with tears streaming down my face brought upon by just the sound of the trailer, I cannot say. But I can say that I never walked out. This may sound like a small point to most people, but it's huge to me. It is largely my resolve that has carried me this far.

As challenging as the trailers were, watching a full-length movie became an exercise in frustration. Mindful of what I know now, it's hard to follow a plot line when you have no recall of the verbal dialogue that took place on the movie screen a mere 5 minutes earlier. As I was unable to hold onto the spoken words, movie watching became an exercise in merely watching pictures. The more colorful and engaging the pictures were, the more apt I was to have a favorable opinion of the movie. I found The Lorax particularly wonderful as the imagery, the 3D textures and vibrant colors were most wonderful indeed. Though I would be hard pressed to tell you anything about the plot line, I did enjoy the colorful experience of that particular flick.

Then came *The Artist.*

It was January 2012 and I was chugging my way through my post-impact life as best I could. Trailers for The Artist showed a silent screen theme. Little did I know that the actual movie was a silent film.

A few minutes into the movie, once we both realized that there was no dialogue, Sarah leaned quietly into my side and asked if I wanted to leave. A quiet left to right shake of my head sealed our fate for the rest of this particular date night. As there was virtually no spoken dialogue for the entire movie, it was sheer action with subtitles that defined that night's experience.

Truth be told, it was by far, the best movie I had seen since my accident. The reason was simple: I was not relying on any verbal queues to understand the plot. Take away the verbal component and effectively my ability to understand content was close to my pre-accident level. Simply put, I watched, rather than listened to the dialogue. And as such, I understood it. As you've seen over and over, brain injury is quite fascinating indeed.

But that still did not take away the fact that I was compromised and that a leading neurologist had diagnosed me as permanently disabled. The implications were stunning. On a professional level, this was close to unacceptable as conversational recall was vital to my ability to run my business. On a personal level, the consequences were even direr. Lost was the ability to have a meaningful back and forth dialogue. Conversations had been reduced to short sentences that were almost immediately forgotten.

Hindsight has offered me so much clarity about this part of my journey. Clarity only comes with time and in the case of my unexpected diagnosis, it took months for me to see it in any kind of perspective.

What the doctor gave me that day was a snapshot of EXACTLY where I was at the time of my testing. Like looking at a single frame of a movie, it reveals a lot, but doesn't show much about the bigger picture.

Yes, I was quite damaged and severely compromised at the time of the testing. I have never doubted the validity of the testing. In fact, it played connect-the-dots with many of the challenges that I had experienced.

What it did not reveal, however, was that I was on a road and not at a final resting point. It did not let me know what future gains I was to make, and was not a real indicator as to what my future would hold.

As you've read already, my biggest gains came months after the neuropsychological testing. Those gains have profoundly impacted the quality of my life for the better. They were gains that were both unexpected in terms of how quickly they occurred, yet fully expected in light of my commitment to get well.

If your own journey involves any type of testing, please be mindful that a single snapshot does not take into consideration what the future will hold. Neural plasticity is a wonderful, amazing and little understood part of the healing process as the brain finds new ways to do what used to be familiar. It continues to this day.

Early on, I shared my vivid recall of the accident and let you know of an unexpected revelation regarding that recall. I was able to paint a very clear picture, with stunning clarity, of the events immediately following my accident.

Or so I thought.

As my neurologist asked me to describe methodically what had unfolded on that fated day, he asked me if I had ever lost consciousness.

I answered a hale and hearty no. How could I have been knocked out cold? I was able to recall "Supermanning" through the air. I could describe the thud of hitting the ground like it was just yesterday. Dialogue with the first responders still can echo through my very being if I bring myself back to that day mentally. No, unconsciousness was not part of the events of the day.

Then he asked me what the first thing was that I saw when I was on the ground, battered and broken. Not understanding the path this astute doctor was leading me down, I shared that I was surrounded by people. Some were crying, others trying to comfort me, others on cell phones. I was surrounded by a small crowd.

And then he dropped the bomb.

"Do you think they just materialized there?"

He had trumped my perceived recall with undisputable reason and logic. He went on to share some common-sense points. Points like the fact that it would take time for a crowd to gather. That during the time it took the crowd to coalesce around me, I laid there on Main Street, knocked out stone cold unconscious, as my brain put together a plausible scenario of events to present to me upon wakening.

The doctor continued on with the fact that it takes a bit of time from the actual creating of the memory until it is laid down in permanent memory. Any memories that I had in the moments before my accident had not yet made it to my own internal hard drive and were lost.

Had I taken a lie detector test at any time up to that great revelation, I would have stated with unwavering confidence that I never lost consciousness. I would have passed the lie detector test with flying colors.

Such is the power of the human brain to attempt to make sense of that which makes no sense; to create reason out of chaos. Yet again, like waves of reality crashing on the beach that my life had become, I sat in stunned awe, my jaw most likely yet again hitting my chest.

Chapter 16

My Daily Life

On more than one occasion, I've sat back and contemplated just how much life has changed since I was thrust into this new dimension of reality. Many of the changes you've already read about. From developing new ways to live with my newfound life changes, to working on accepting that I am now running a new kind of marathon, my day-to-day life in one sense mirrors my pre-accident life.

Daily I wake up, attend to the life responsibilities in front of me as best I can, do all I can to balance work, home, career, and personal relationships like most anyone, brain injured or not.

My smaller circle of closer friends knows of my struggles and I will be eternally grateful to have a handful of friends who have opted to stick by me. They will never know that they are a big part of why I am even alive today.

On the outside, things look very much like they did before my injury. Ask many brain injury survivors what three words can really stir up emotions, and you will almost universally hear the words, "you look normal."

While my body has healed, my soul, my very spirit, that part of me that makes me who I am, remains forever changed. And many of those changes are so wondrously unexpected.

I am able to connect with people in a way that I was never able to before my injury. Gone is any sense of being apart from humanity. We are all members of the same human family; we all have the right to be here, and no one, regardless of skin color, ethnicity, and degree of brain injury or otherwise are any better or worse in my world. I was never one to let prejudices define my life before I was injured; there is simply a new level of connectivity to everything.

Prior to my accident, I had two speeds: overdrive and stop. I was either full-tilt out rocking and rolling through life or I was asleep. My world was very black and white. I now have a deep appreciation for the grays of life. My respect for all things living is right off the charts. Again, this is not really a deviation from who I was before the accident, it is more like an enhancement of my core values. So completely unexpected and at times wondrous, it's an unexpected gift from this whole experience.

My love for music has been rekindled and I no longer "hear" music like I once did. Rather, I "feel" music at a soul level that I never envisioned possible. Until I read about music therapy helping Gabby Giffords learn to speak again, I never gave much thought to the added benefit of listening my MP3 player for two hours a day.

While my ability to speak was abruptly compromised a few months after my accident, my ability to really enjoy and be part of the music I listened to daily was never compromised. Daily I would cycle thirty miles or more and quietly hum along with my favorite musical artists.

Not once did I give thought to the fact that this daily musical exercise could actually have been part of my brain's process of reconstructing itself. Yet today I am able, most of the time, to articulate my thoughts and ideas, albeit at a pace a bit slower than before, in such a way that most would not even know I had a speech impediment.

I look at the brain with wonder and amazement as there are times that it knows what is best for me before I do.

Always one to love nature, when Sarah and I often find ourselves at the local seashore, or perhaps hiking through a New Hampshire meadow, I am now often the one to stop when a wildflower catches my eye and marvel for time longer than I ever thought possible at the simple beauty of a flower. I am left feeling connected in what amounts to a Disney-like circle of life kind of way.

No longer do I focus on the destination as I once did. Rather, akin to savoring a wonderful meal, I take smaller bites out of the day's experiences and savor them in a way that I never thought possible.

As you've seen, life is not without challenges, many of them major. But there are silver linings to many of the clouds, linings that I never looked for.

Like those wiser than I will ever be, I am careful of where I focus my attention. I try to be ever-mindful of the power of my mind to define my reality. If I chose to focus on my daily challenges, living in constant mourning for the life I once had, I rob myself of the ability to enjoy the life that I have.

In many respects, I am living my second life. It is such a blessing to have the experience of living two separate, yet so interconnected lives; so few have had the privilege of doing so. Yet, sometimes I am blindsided and overwhelmed by the intensity of it all.

This tale started with a chance meeting with a young man. Close to two years later our paths crossed again. It's only fitting that he become part of the closing to this part of my tale.

A recent High School graduation ceremony I attended brought it all full circle. Sometimes life rocks you at times you least expect it, and the rug gets pulled out from under you when you never even knew you were standing on it.

Such was the case on our local High School's graduation day in 2012.

Sarah and I were at Salem High School attending my stepson's graduation. The day was about as perfect as you could ever expect: blue skies, puffy clouds, light breeze and a huge amount of positive energy, smiles and photo taking.

We sat side-by-side in the bleachers watching the kids accept diplomas, listening to families cheer and watching the contraband beach balls bounce across the field.

Lost in a bit of fun picture taking, Sarah leaned over, pointed to one of the kids and said two words that redefined my day.

"That's _____," she whispered quietly, referring to the young driver who hit me.

The rush of emotion was shocking, stunning, intense, and close to indescribable. Had I been standing, I would have come close to collapsing. (But you can't really collapse while sitting, can you?)

Tears streamed as my waterworks went from zero to 6 in a millisecond. It was like every emotion I felt in the last 19 months came out all at once. I'd never experienced anything like that in over half a century of riding this rock.

Leaning into Sarah's side, I clutched her arm to stay upright and fought with Herculean force to regain my composure. It was the special day for someone else. There was no need for my "stuff" to taint the day for everyone else. Later, Sarah said that as soon as she let me know it was the young man who hit me who walked by, I was immediately "diminished," my confidence was instantly gone and my lights went out.

Apt choice of a word: diminished.

It was only later that clarity came. It was a PTSD event in its truest sense. How did I feel, seeing the one who drove into me? Who damaged my brain? Who left me forever changed? There was no anger. No resentment. No hatred. No ill will.

I quietly wished him a full and happy life.

The realization that I still carry wounds most will never see came full circle again. And yes, I snapped his picture. As I sat there in the bleachers thinking about him, and that Fated, awful day, I found myself hoping that he wasn't thinking about it too.

In all likelihood, he wasn't.

Not a day goes by where the overwhelming reality of how my life has changed hits me like a brick. It's shocking. Unexpected. Unplanned for. When I was a young man, planning out the course of my life, this was not supposed to be part of the plan.

Or maybe it was...

A hard-hitting reality check happened on wintery January night in 2012. The type of reality check that made me question, not for the first time, if my fate was determined long before I showed up for my own accident.

As sleep remains problematic at best with my ongoing PTSD nightmares, at the suggestion of one of my doctors I try to get in to bed at a pretty consistent timeframe that will let me get 8 or so hours of sleep.

If you told me a couple of years ago that I would have a bedtime ritual that included chamomile tea, no TV watching and a period of winding down with some meditation, I would have laughed heartily. A couple of nightmares can help you to rethink this. Kick it up a notch to over a year of 2-3 nightmares a week and you'll do just about anything to try to sleep. In fact, had I been told to do handstands for 15 minutes before bed to get relief from the nightmares, I would have done so in a heartbeat.

Having completed my nightly sleep ritual, I hunkered down for another night. Long gone was the anticipation of restful sleep. If a night passes without a hair-raising nightmare, I count myself lucky.

Then it happened.

3:15 AM. The house shook. It shook so hard, it felt like I was going to fall out of bed. Sarah and I sat bolt upright. Her "mom gears" were instantly activated and she checked on all the kids. The children were nestled all snug in their beds, though I've been told that Christmas had already passed.

Voices echoed through our yard. Peering out the bedroom window, I saw someone standing adjacent to our side yard talking on a cell phone. Grabbing a pair of shoes, I bolted out of the house and into a scene of complete and utter chaos.

It seems that a younger driver, only 21, had taken the curve on the road outside our house just a bit too fast, failed to compensate for the icy road conditions of that night, and hit a telephone pole in our yard at full speed. His impact was hard enough to snap the utility pole in half.

Obviously in shock, he was on his cell phone babbling and not making much sense. As I asked if he was OK, a young woman came into view. Looking not more than 18, she stood by the car, shell-shocked and bleeding profusely from a head injury. Her blond hair matted with blood, she stood by the roadside screaming.

It took all of a 3 count for me to bolt back to the house.

Sarah was on the phone with 9-1-1 in under a minute.

Knowing that help was on the way, I headed back outside. Steam was pouring from the front of the car and the utility pole that was struck tipped precariously. Eyes scanning this unexpected winter landscape, it was made even more eerie as the ungodly screaming continued. I let the young man know that help was on the way and prudently fell back into the shadows. Not knowing whether alcohol was involved, I deemed it wise to step back.

You know already that my accident was only a block from the Main Street Fire Station. My home is only a few blocks from one of the other fire stations in town. In what felt like only a minute or two, fire and rescue vehicles flooded the street with flashing lights and spotlights. I stood on my back deck watching the events unfold with tears streaming down my face, my body wracked with soft sobs.

Based on my own experience, I don't handle high emotion like I used to. In fact, for months after the accident, when the rescue vehicles would leave the fire station down the street and come wailing by our home, I would stop dead in my tracks, frozen in time, until they passed. More often than not, my eyes still well up in tears when I hear an ambulance.

I watched the rescue personnel strap the young girl to the gurney, load her in a waiting ambulance, and whisk her away. I said a quiet prayer for all involved and went back in the house, never expecting to see them again.

Then Fate intervened again.

A week later, while working in my home office, the front doorbell rang. I answered the door to a couple of young kids and asked if I could help them. There was no familiarity to their faces, no recognition.

The young man spoke first.

"We were the ones involved in the accident in front of your house last week," he said with a bit of trepidation, "and we wanted to thank you."

It was at that time that I noticed the face of the girl standing beside him. She wore extra large sunglasses to hide her badly bruised face. What she could not hide, however, were the three lines of sutures that went from her hairline to her glasses. More stitches than I could count adorned her face.

"The doctors said that it was the fact that she got help so fast that prevented even more damage to her."

He went on to say that she was initially taken to a local hospital. Once her condition was assessed, she was taken immediately to a Boston area hospital based on the severity of her head injury. She had a brain injury.

Now it was my turned to be shell-shocked. Here on my front door step was a young man who was doing the exact same thing that I did after my accident. He was taking the time to offer a sincere and heartfelt thank you to someone who came to his aid. Rather than being the Giver of Thanks, that day found me the recipient of appreciation unexpected.

I choked back tears. I do that a lot these days. I also shared briefly about my own accident. We shared a moment as we all regaled the local fire and rescue folks with well deserved compliments.

My eyes lingered on her head injury. Raw and obscene, her young face looked like it was scarred with profanity. It was unnatural. Young people, people younger than my own sons, were not supposed to get brain injuries.

But they do.

Every 21 seconds, someone in America gets a brain injury. In the time it's taken you to read this far, it's a safe bet to say that there have been dozens of brain injurics.

America's silent epidemic? You tell me.

I wished them both well as they left and offered an invitation to stop by at any time to let me know how they were doing. I closed the front door, retreated back to my office and called Sarah. It took a few minutes for me to get beyond the high emotion and even begin to tell her what had just transpired.

More emotion. Even more tears.

The enormity of it all came raging in again. Here was I, trying to rebuild my life... a life with a brain injury, and what comes knocking at my door? A newly brain injured member of the human family.

What are the odds of this unfolding of events?

Suffice to say, any consideration of productive work was gone for the rest of that day. I took my afternoon bike ride and did a lot of thinking. It was not the first time that I wondered whether this was all part of a grander design; a plan for my life that was set before I was even born. I wondered about my own destiny.

Again.

Chapter 17

Metamorphosis

As a young child, I was always one to shun the main-stream. Not only was this tolerated, it was actually encouraged.

My father has long been one of the best teachers I've had in my life. He did not teach by dictation or rule. No, his was more of an illustrative type of teaching. As a young man, he showed me by living example the importance of living an honorable life.

Daily he would "suit up and show up" for life. Looking back to my life as a child, he would go to work Mondays through Fridays, pay the bills, and do his best to always do the right thing. This was never done for attention, mind you. It was simply the right thing to do, no questions asked.

In the mid 1970's, my dad went through what he has openly called his mid-life crisis. He quit his long-standing job in the aerospace industry, grew out his hair and beard and proceeded to do... well... nothing.

Thankfully, that phase didn't last for long, my mom let him get it out of his system, his employer gratefully took him back on board, and we, as a family, barely missed a heartbeat.

It was during this time that I first noticed a quote hanging on the wall of his bedroom. It was another of those coincidences that leaves me feeling that there is really a Grand Plan in life. The quote was by Henry David Thoreau who has been a literary inspiration to me for the better part of my adult life.

At the age of 12, however, I hadn't a clue about this great visionary.

The quote that hung upon Dad's wall is a concept that should be taught in every school as it is the epitome of tolerance for ones' fellow man.

> "If a man does not keep pace with his companions, perhaps it is because he hears a different drummer. Let him step to the music which he hears, however measured or far away." ~ Henry David Thoreau

Here were the words that defined, at least in part, the reality of life as I knew it. Individualism was not only accepted, it was a requisite. Uniqueness was not uncommon. Rather, it was the norm in what amounted to the ultimate oxymoron.

And we come full circle to butterflies and metamorphosis.

For many years, while my pre-adolescent peers were out catching baseballs, I spent my time catching butterflies. No folly here. I had a legitimate child-like wonderment of these amazing and graceful creatures.

In fields and meadows from New Hampshire to Maine and back to Massachusetts, I quietly stalked my prey. My ever-present net in hand, nimble as only a child can be, I patiently waited for the next new discovery to flutter by.

I had butterfly books, butterfly cases, and watched any television show that even remotely had to do with these graceful flyers. When a new catch would come my way, I would preserve them in the types of cases that the entomologists use. You've no doubt seen them in museums with glass in front and cotton batten pressing the butterflies into the glass. My childhood specimens were preserved to this degree of scientific accuracy.

Even today, on the wall of my office hangs one of those cases from my childhood. A Luna moth forever frozen in eternity next to a Tiger Swallowtail; a Viceroy butterfly the constant and silent companion to a Polyphemus moth.

They have survived the passage of time. Mounted perhaps 40 or more years ago, they are a vivid testimonial to my early mounting skills.

It's worth noting that today such an activity would not mesh with my world. I deem all life to be sacred. Other than an errant wasp, most any bug that is lucky enough to get into our home is not squashed. No, they are gently caught and released back into the Wild.

Such was the bliss of youth however, as I had no real awareness that the vital life force that flows through all of us also flowed through my colorful captives.

The entire process of metamorphosis captivated me. Here were caterpillars that had no real beauty, it seemed. They had no awareness of their future and lived in blissful ignorance of what was to become of them.

Chomping on leaves and growing day-by-day, earth-bound by circumstance and not choice, the freedom of flight would be beyond their comprehension.

Yet fly they would. Gracefully. Beautifully. As completely transformed beings.

So it has become with my brain injury. My pre-injury life was akin to the life of the caterpillar. Moving day-by-day, earthbound and living a familiar routine, I had no idea, no comprehension, no way of knowing how much I would change. The veil that blocks our ability to see beyond the moment blocked any inkling of what the future would hold.

Like the caterpillar heading into his cocoon for a long period of darkness and change, so were the months after my accident. My world got immensely small and dark. The light of day was almost entirely blotted out but, within the confines of my own cocoon, I was changing. Like the butterfly, I would be the last to know.

I emerged from my darkness forever changed and vastly different than the being I was before my accident.

Many years ago I read a story that I thought was about a butterfly. As I grow in life experience, I now see that it's really not about a butterfly at all. Rather, it is about the purely human requirement for adversity in life and the ability of life's hardships to not only strengthen us, but to define who we are.

The Butterfly

A man found a cocoon of a butterfly. One day a small opening appeared. He sat and watched the butterfly for several hours as it struggled to force its body through that little hole.

Then it seemed to stop making any progress. It appeared as if it had gotten as far as it could and it could go no farther.

Then the man decided to help the butterfly, so he took a pair of scissors and snipped off the remaining bit of the cocoon. The butterfly emerged easily. But it had a swollen body and small, shriveled wings.

The man continued to watch the butterfly because he expected that, at any moment, the wings would enlarge and expand to be able to support the body, which would contract in time.

Neither happened! In fact, the butterfly spent the rest of its life crawling around with a swollen body and shriveled wings. It was never able to fly.

What the man in his kindness and haste did not understand was that the restricting cocoon and the struggle required for the butterfly to get through the tiny opening were God's way of forcing fluid from the body of the butterfly into its wings so that it would be ready for flight once it achieved its freedom from the cocoon.

Sometimes struggles are exactly what we need in our life. If God allowed us to go through our life without any obstacles it would cripple us. We would not be as strong as what we could have been. And we could never fly.

No longer earth-bound, I have new wings. New insight and new perspectives define my reborn sense of self.

Yes, the process of emerging was difficult. Slowly, as I broke free of my own personal cocoon, I knew things were different. While I lacked the physical wings to soar, my spirit was free. I had come through the most difficult chapter of my life thus far.

I am forever changed. There is no going back.

But today I look to a future that is brighter than anything I ever thought possible. My compassion for those who struggle has increased ten-fold. My experience has humbled me. Lessons unasked for have redefined me.

As I soar through my new reality, I have been privileged to meet others who now soar as well.

My simple wish for you is this: If you find yourself in a dark place with no light or hope, please remember that often this is a monumental turning point.

As the future becomes the present and time passes by, you will soar again, freer than you ever thought possible.

Peace,

~David

Life After Dark

Perhaps the most unexpected and unpredictable part of this journey has been dealing with Post Traumatic Stress Disorder. Secondary to my brain injury, my PTSD has added a new element of surrealism to my journey.

Some of the effects have come and gone. Though it was a mere thirty days or so after my accident that I hobbled back onto my trusty bike again, it took me months to be able to bike beyond the confines of my neighborhood. In fact, it was close to six months post-impact that I was able to cross a street with a yellow line. Fear kept me close to home.

Never one to be shy of being out and about, I have a limited ability to be out in crowds for long. My life is far from reclusive. But being around lots of people for more than a short while leaves me exhausted like never before.

Yes, I startle with unexpected intensity these days. Come up behind me quietly and say "boo" and you'll see a pair of shoes on the ground and not much more. I am told this is normal in light of my near death experience.

But it's the nightmares that continue to be the most intense after-effect of all of this. At the time of this writing, I am well into year two of my new life, yet this past week alone has seen three nights of abject terror.

I have learned to live with it, though it's tough on Sarah. Yes, I am a writer and have been since long before my accident, so how do I cope with my night terrors? You most likely know the answer by now... I write.

Never one for sensationalism, in my dreams I have suffered most every manner of death and discomfort imaginable. From dismemberment to being disemboweled, from drowning to horrific car wrecks, my night dreams are as richly textured as reality.

Strike that; they are more like reality on steroids. Colors are more vibrant, textures are richer, and my dream pain is more exquisite than anything I have experienced in my waking reality.

From a short stint of doctor-prescribed medication to over a year of intense therapy, I've done all I can to make my life more livable.

Yet death stalks me to this day. I hold out hope that this chapter of my life will someday move to the back seat. If I lose hope, I lose everything.

My intent is not to close with any type of morbidity. I am alive. Though at times slightly challenging, I am so much better off than I could have been. But to paint a real picture of life after brain injury and all that it encompasses, it is a personal requisite that I share just a few of my after-dark experiences.

You are about to meet a few of my night time friends. *The Voodoo Queen* has made numerous stops in my dreams since my accident. She is a repeat visitor to my land of horrors. In *The Wrestler*, you'll meet one of two of the unnamed cast of characters that haunt me. *My Other Life* is a tale unto itself as this was a waking nightmare - the entire tale came to me while cycling one day. Riding along, I listened to my mind tell me this unfamiliar tale. I dashed home and penned it before its memory evaporated.

Welcome to my life after dark...

The Wrestler

Never having wrestled in a ring before, it was odd. The spotlights lit up the ring but shielded my ability to see the audience. Whether there was one or many, I knew it not. Odder still... I was wrestling a man with no arms.

Casting his body from one end of the ring to the other, he dashed at me, charged me, head butted me, and ran for the safety of the ropes. And he had my face.

Never having lived as an amputee, it was odd being in a wrestling ring with no arms, yet, there I found myself. I was not able to discern who my nemesis was. Unlike my shattered state, he was wholly whole with both arms intact. I knew I had to fight hard or die. The odds were clearly against me. I was not going to die again in yet another Fractured Fairy Tale.

I could feel his vice-like arms around my neck. With no arms, I had no way to fight back. Writhing and squirming, I knew that I was beaten; that my luck was about to run out. No mere victory for my foe, he was intent on killing me.

I could feel his sweat. No arms, he squirmed like one about to die. But why shouldn't he? I was about to kill him. Pulling my arms tighter, I heard the first crack as his spine snapped. Pulling just a bit harder, it cracked again and I knew my job was done.

I let the lifeless body fall to the floor.

Feeling my neck crack the first time, I knew the End was coming. The second crack sealed my Fate.

And then it happened...

From two unique entities in the ring came one as I abruptly realized that I was not two. No duality of beings here. I was alone in the ring, falling to the floor, my own arms wrapped around my neck as I had just snapped my own neck.

Truth be told, night time now terrifies me. Doing all I can to overcome, the battle is fought nightly.

No more sweet dreams, only endless carnage.

Voodoo Queen

She sat across from me, a stark wooden table and two rickety chairs the only adornments of a room I could not see. She would not look at me. Her hands were working furiously as she spoke in unfamiliar tongues. It was clear that this was some type of incantation, the purpose of which would reveal itself soon enough.

I watched in endless fascination as her hands shape shifted over a small plate, animal parts in various states of decay being pulled apart by long bony fingers.

Just us two: Me, a lost soul, and the Voodoo Lady, attentive to the task at hand.

The incantation stopped.

She sat up and revealed a face that was a hideous mask of pleasure. And she laughed. Laughed a laugh that would make any brave soul want to run and cowl.

And in a heartbeat, I knew what her spell was cast for.

At that moment, I felt a second soul move into my physical body. Like trying on a suit, my mind felt a new presence within the body I have heretofore lived in as the sole occupant. The symbolism is stunningly surreal.

And I screamed.

And she cackled on.

And the new resident of my body tried to push my own soul to the side, to kick me to the curb.

On occasion, I can reach beyond the veil that separates the waking mind from sleeping mind. On a few occasions, I am able to call out, through my terror, three words that are like a life ring to my suffering.

Sarah, unaware of where my mind has gone on any given night hears me yell those simple words of quiet desperation...

"WAKE ME UP!"

And she tries, as best she can, to pull me back from the abyss. To bring me home and let me know none of it is real. Not so with the Voodoo Lady. Vocal cords cut; I can't utter my new distress call. I am at her mercy.

My Other Life

March 24, 1824

I swear that all I write today is truth. This I swear in the name of our King, George III. As sure as the ink flows from the feathered pen in my shaking hand, the events I am about to tell you came to pass. As my memories fade fast, I fear that failing to put quill to paper, I will forget, that like so much of my past life, these events will fade.

It's hard to believe that a mere four months ago, I was a Duke in northern Britain serving our Royal King George III. The Duchess Sarah by my side, we lived an enviable life: Stables of fine horses, a thousand head of cattle grazing and servants whose quarters were the envy of the townspeople. Dinner nightly on fine porcelain imported by my brother, heir to the East India Trading Company, we ate from the finest of china, our flatware alone worth more than a common miller or cooper would earn in a lifetime.

Never would I have expected life to turn about as it did starting on a fine November day last fall. The hounds, following the scent of a fox, darted straight into a hollow between two stands of tall pines. So engrossed in the hunt was I that I failed to see the lower bough of the pine before I struck it. Thrown from my mare, I landed hard on the English earth, knowing not how my life was about to change.

My footman assisted me back on my steed, though I have little memory of this. I have no need to doubt his word as he served me honorably for nigh of twenty years. His period of indenturement close to complete, it was my intent to bequeath him a parcel of land 200 furlongs square, but alas, all this has changed.

Little recall do I have of the days following my accident. But it was at that time that the nightmares began. Writhing in bed as one possessed by a daemonic force, I cried out in mortal terror. The Duchess Sarah by my side, lost and bewildered at my night time torments. In our hamlet, word traveled fast.

"The Duke has madness about him," townspeople whispered behind shuttered windows as they drained their pints of ale. The Monsignor was notified and an ensuing investigation saw me accused as a witch. What else would explain the night time ranting, the screams, the speaking in tongues and my memories of a future I've never seen?

Why, in one such dream, the Devil himself appeared. While he spoke to me in soft whispers, one of his minions, catlike in ability, climbed a nearby tree. Tethered at his waistcoat with what appeared to be a ships rigging, the evil minion danced his way, defying the laws that hold us to earth, in an easy sidestep up the tree, akin to an insect. Tied to the rope, by their necks, were four young people, their pupils dark with wide terror, knowing not their fate.

High above the ground, the Devil's servant jumped, pulling the line taught. I watched in fascination as events unforeseen unfolded, and listened in rapt horror as the rope, pulled close to its breaking point, snapped the necks of the Innocents, their bodies falling into a heap like mere cordwood. Try as she might, the Duchess Sarah was unable to comfort me after that episode and I stared wide eyed at the canopy above our bed for the remainder of the night.

Am I blessed or cursed to be where I am now?

The formal inquisition by the Monsignor saw me accused, tried and convicted of witchcraft. Truth be told, if I had heard the same ranting by one of my own servants I would have at the least, thought him mad, and more likely possessed as well. I do not blame the Monsignor. Sentenced to hang at the Gallows, I was. Located behind the Parrish Church, I was to hang at sunset on a Saturday. Hanging never took place on Sundays as that is the Lord's Day. Had it not been for the fact that my brothers son was in direct service of the King, I surely would not have lived to tell this tale.

A harsh choice was proffered: To die by hanging or to relinquish my life, my Dukedom, and all my earthly possessions and be vanquished to the New World. By now, you know my choice.

As I dip my pen again and resume writing this tale, we are thirty seven days to sea. The shipmen tell me I am in an infirmary, but I've never seen an infirmary with bars and a locked door. More like a brig, it is. The former Duchess Sarah was given the choice to hang or to join me in exile. As our love is undying, she is joining me, hoping a trip across the Sea will find my daemons left in Britain. I have not the heart to tell her that I still awaken, most of the time well after moonrise, writhing in fear and covered in sweat. The captain of this vessel, a fair and honest soldier of the King's Army, allows Sarah to bring me bread and water once daily. Occasionally, she sneaks me a bowl of gruel, though I well know that the days she does that, she herself goes hungry. Such is the bond of our love. She would give all for me, and I her.

Not all my dreams are of terrors and satanic forces. Last week, I dreamed I was sitting in front of a window on a small stand. It sat upon a desk of mahogany. My dreams are like that, you know, richly textured and lifelike. In my dreams eye, I could see pictures in the window that sat upon my desk. Stranger still, my hands were hovering over what looked like a box for the tools of a craftsman. As my hands hovered over the box, words appeared, as if by magic, within the lighted window on my desk. I dare not share this dream with anyone as my lunacy will be confirmed. Hear tell, it is just as early to meet the hangman in the New World as it is the Olde. In fact, though it's been over a century since the witches of Salem met their due demise, I hope to not add to the list on the hangman's roster. The witches of Salem were true witches. I, however, am merely the victim of an equestrian accident. No more, no less.

Why, just last night, I dreamt of my name on a headstone, Sarah's headstone by my side, on the hillside of an unfamiliar land. My hope is that this is not portend of evil; a sign of events that shall come to pass; A window into an unfamiliar future.

In the name of my Lord and Savior Jesus Christ, and in my undying gratitude to King George III for sparing my life, I remain,

David Webster

March 24, 1824

"Welcome to my Nightmare..."

The world was in a post apocalyptic state. It was survive or die. Walking down Main Street of what was left of a small-town American town, they approached me.

"If you want to pass this way alive, you'll need to talk to Her."

Against my will, I was strong-armed into a small shanty shack. Rough unfinished pine boards made up the wall. The walls and floor were uneven. Through the cracks between the boards, a monochrome world existed, devoid of any life. A fire orange sun on the horizon casted the only visible color.

The shack, reminiscent of what you might expect a 19th century miners' shack to look like, had 2 small rooms: One room was full of decimated, lost souls, sunken eyes, and the stench of humanity; the other room hidden from view by a small doorway.

Shoved by hands unseen, I was thrust into the second room. Void of furnishings, save one: a bent and broken table against the wall. Void of people, save one. Behind the table She sat. Looking like an unkempt palm reader, she beckoned me over.

"If you want to live, you need to play the game..." I more felt her words than heard them. They resonated in my soul. I knew as surely as I write this that if failed her test, I would die.

Bony hands in tattered clothes worked a shell game. Sliding left, sliding right... charms that may well have been human bones nestled under the shells.

My heart read hers. I knew she was toying with me, with my life. She had no intention of letting me go. I was a mere insect in her web. When she was done playing and the novelty that was me wore off, my Doom awaited. She would kill me.

And then it happened and I seized the moment. One of the shells slid off the table. As She leaned over to snatch it up in her bony fingers, I chose my moment.

My feet were clad in dust covered boots and I know this for one reason only.

As she leaned down, I raised my boot and let it come down on her neck with all the force I had. I knew a second chance awaited me not. It was not the sound so much that bothered me. Rather, it was the feeling of the bones breaking under my foot that was most troubling. I knew in a heartbeat that her neck was snapped. Her body tumbled off the chair and fell to the floor.

Realizing that time was not my friend, I left her lair, stumbled into the other room and looked at the lost souls that returned my hollow stare.

"You are free of Her!" I proclaimed like a post-apocalyptic abolitionist. "You can go now..."

But they moved not. Their eyes weren't staring at me, or even through me. They were watching what was happening behind me.

Catching a sudden motion out of the corner of my eye, I spun around. The corpse of the Gypsy woman crossed the room in supernatural speed, covering a 15 foot distance in under a second.

Blink. She is across the room.

Blink. She is a foot from me.

A pen knife with a 4" blade in her bony hand dripped with blood. The souls behind me letting me know there was no escape.

And her corpse... The impact of my foot severed her head. She stood there, knife thrust toward my heart, no eyes to see, but knowing her knife would hit its mark.

And I stood there. Knowing I was about to die.

And I screamed.

And I screamed under my blankets. Sarah pulled me back to reality. Sweat soaked and trembling, I opened my eyes and scanned the room. Looking for Her.

Hoping She wasn't able, by some supernatural ability, to leap from my nightmare to my bedroom.

I trembled. Until the arms of Sarah held me close and let me know it was only another dream.

Yet another dream...

The Story Continues

When I started writing this book, I envisioned a book purely about moving forward through life after suffering a brain injury. But, it's been so much more. Through the process of looking back on my life since my injury, looking back at the triumphs, the hardships, the joys and the tears, I can see that these life lessons transcend brain injury.

The real lessons I have learned are too many to share in one book. In fact, I am still learning. The value of real friends in times of crisis, having someone's hand to hold when the path ahead is dark and uncertain, knowing deep inside that against all odds, life will indeed go on. These concepts are not unique to my journey.

My hope for you is simple: No matter your current circumstance, may you find joy in the journey, friends to stand by you, and an unwavering, if not child-like faith in the goodness of the Universe.

Thank you for walking with me for but a few steps in my own life's journey.

Meet the Author

Many people, even those who know me best, often ask what I do. Rather than bore someone with the ins and outs of my day-to-day life, I often just say, "'I create things."

Yes, there is a certain mystique with a response like that. This all-encompassing statement is meant to reach beyond my professional life and actually touches all aspects of my life. Yes, I am a nationally published author. I create thoughts and images in the minds of my readers by the words I lay down on paper.

But that is just the tip of my own personal iceberg.

Professionally, I create with the written word, graphic artwork, and a wide range of other mediums in the daily world of running my company. Personally, I create as well. I work to create and recreate a safe and sacred space in our home. I create relationships and meaningful friendships.

But these days, the creation of a new life, a life after brain injury, is the main focus of my life. Long before my injury, I had a voice that carried. My written work has seen worldwide distribution over the last decade. I now use my new voice to cast a spotlight on America's silent epidemic: Traumatic Brain Injury.

My hope is that you now have a better understanding of what life is like after sustaining a brain injury. Watch for my next title, *The Brain Injury Handbook*. This compelling guide will offer insight and practical real-world information to help survivors navigate through life after a brain injury.

If you have found this book to be insightful and helpful as you journey through your own life, please take a moment to review it on Amazon.com. This will help others to benefit for the message of hope and recovery I share.

To continue following my journey, please visit my blog at www.DavidsNewLife.com